About the Pul

BPP Learning Media is dedicated to supporting aspiring professionals with top quality learning material. BPP Learning Media's commitment to success is shown by our record of quality, innovation and market leadership in paper-based and e-learning materials. BPP Learning Media's study materials are written by professionally-qualified specialists who know from personal experience the importance of top quality materials for success.

Reaching your Goal

The process of applying to medical school can be a somewhat long and arduous process but the rewards of a career within Medicine are infinite. BPP Learning Media and BPP University College School of Health are committed to supporting aspiring and current doctors to progress their career through our comprehensive range of books, personal development courses and degree programmes. I often say there is no other vocation that provides such breadth and depth of career options for the individual to follow and specialise in. Whether it is the fast paced nature of the A&E department or the measured environment of Pathology, there is something for everyone.

There is no greater privilege than being responsible for leading the treatment of patients and sharing in their recovery. There are few other careers that provide such diversity on a daily basis. A passion for helping others, clear communication skills especially empathy, excellent team working and leadership qualities as well as the ability to strike a work-life balance are all skills that an accomplished doctor should possess.

The decision to follow a career in Medicine is something that should not be taken lightly and you should undertake careful research to ensure it really is for you. A career in Medicine is not for everyone and I would urge readers to ensure they have undertaken sufficient work experience to gain a balanced insight into what becoming a doctor really entails.

I first began mentoring aspiring medical students seven years ago when it was clear that many individuals were not gaining access to the help and support they required to successfully apply to medical school. It was with this in mind that I embarked on publishing our Entry to Medical School Series to provide a clear insight into the various facets of successfully getting into medical school. Whether it is help with choosing the right medical school , how to prepare an outstanding personal statement or how to succeed in your medical school interview, our comprehensive range of books provide the advice that is so often hard to find.

I would like to take this opportunity to wish you the very best of luck with applying to medical school and hope that you pass on some of the gems of wisdom that you acquire along the way to other aspiring medics.

Matt Green
Series Editor – Entry to Medical School
Medical Publishing Director

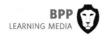

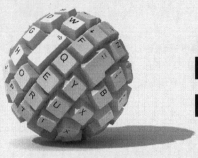

Free Companion Material

Readers can access a comprehensive list of practice interview questions for free online.

To access the above companion material please visit **www.bpp.com/freehealthresources**

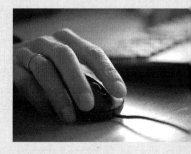

BPP
LEARNING MEDIA

About the Authors

Tony Edgar, MSc, MBBS, FFPH

Tony qualified in Medicine from Newcastle University in 1971. After working as a principal in general practice in north east England, he undertook specialty training in public health in Manchester. In 1990 he was appointed as Director of Public Health in West Lancashire Health Authority; in 1994 he took up the post of Medical Director of the Fosse Health NHS Trust in Leicestershire, and Honorary Lecturer at Leicester University. In 2002 he was elected Fellow of the Faculty of Public Health of the United Kingdom.

Matt Green, BSc (Hons), MPhil

Matt Green has spent the last six years directly helping over 5,000 individuals successfully apply to medical school. It is with this extensive experience in mind that Matt has written this book to help prospective medical students prepare for the interview as part of their application to medical school.

Matt and Tony are keen to share their respective experiences in supporting applicants to medical school, in preparing fully for the interview and to reach their full potential.

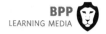

Acknowledgements

I would like to say thank you to Alice for always being there over the years and for encouraging me to be myself.

I would also like to extend a warm thank you to Tony for continuing to be involved in this book. It has been a pleasure and a privilege to work alongside you.

Matt Green

We would also like to acknowledge the many applicants who have met with us and shared their experiences with us.

From both Tony and Matt, we wish our readers every success in securing your place at medical school.

Good Luck.

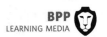

Preface

What is Medicine?

To study Medicine at university is to learn about the science of the human body in health and disease, and then to apply that knowledge when caring for patients and working alongside colleagues. To practise Medicine is to combine effective communication with practical skills.

Over the last several years we have gained considerable experience in helping prospective medical students with all stages of their applications.

This has included conducting:

- one day interview workshops, where applicants take part in interactive sessions looking at all aspects of the medical school interview, and
- intensive 'one-to-one' sessions.

This informative guide is intended to help school leaver, graduate and mature applicants in their preparations.

Our goal is to help all candidates seeking to study Medicine at university maximise their chance of selection by enabling them to bring their very best qualities to the medical school interview.

Please use this guide together with advice provided by your school or college, from the Universities and College Admissions Service, and alongside assistance offered by the medical schools themselves.

The most important aspect of your application to medical school, including particularly your performance at interview, is that it fully reflects your own, unique personality.

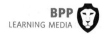

Chapter 1

Background

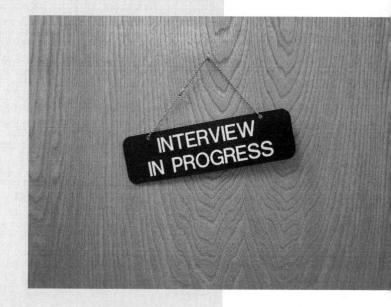

Background

This book is written to help applicants to medical schools in the United Kingdom make the very most of the opportunity given to them when invited for interview. When we talk of 'succeeding' in a medical school interview, we mean that the candidate acquits themselves as well as they possibly can. Of course, the main objective for any applicant is to receive an offer of a place to study Medicine. But even on those occasions when the interview signals that a student is not suited to, or just not ready to study Medicine, the fact that the interview helps the candidate to arrive at that conclusion sooner rather than later comprises a successful outcome to the process – a good purpose will have been served.

It is certainly our experience, and it is entirely understandable, that some students seek assistance in preparing for their interview by inquiring: 'If the interviewer asks me question X, or question Y, what are the right things to say?'

Well, there will be questions asked by panel members which explore matters of factual knowledge, and on those occasions the 'right things to say' are self-evident. However, medical school interview panels are not simply seeking to assess how much one candidate *knows* about a range of issues compared to other candidates.

Panels are determined to challenge candidates, and to take them outside their 'comfort zone'. They are so much more interested in finding out about their personalities: what judgements have they begun to form, and what are their personal values?

It is in this light which we believe that we are simply not in a position to suggest what the right thing is *for you* to say. You will have your own unique personality, and it is this, above all, that the panel is keen to discover.

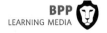

So, it is important to understand at the outset that this book does not provide a set of 'model', right answers to a list of anticipated questions.

However, we will look at frameworks around which potential responses to imagined questions might be constructed, and upon which you can then apply your own individuality.

Our key aim is to enable you to have the confidence to be yourself, to have the self-belief to present your own views, and not to be driven to present comments on the basis simply that you think they will please the panel.

We seek to equip you to engage – at times fluently, and always courteously and carefully – with the interviewers in a style that is wholly your own.

Indeed, based upon our experience over the last several years, we believe that this book can act as a guide whereby you can increase your confidence and self-belief to the point that you will be able to handle anything the interview panel puts to you.

Rather than attempting to provide a collection of answers, we seek to encourage you to adopt what we believe is the *right approach* in preparing your *responses* to the panel's questions.

This approach is founded on two vital principles:

You must prepare to be at ease, to be self-confident, *at all times* during your discussions with the panel.

There will be times when it all feels very straightforward; for example, when you are asked questions exploring your factual knowledge in areas which are of great interest to you.

However, medical school interview panels are very skilled in what they do. And you can depend upon it – they will be very

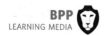

determined to see how you handle the occasions when your fluent responses 'dry up'.

So, yes, it is important to enter the interview with a strong knowledge base. However, it is perhaps even more important that you are equipped to remain calm, courteous and confident when the panel take you outside areas of factual understanding.

Accordingly, good, effective preparation is not based upon cramming as much knowledge upon as many topics as possible.

It is even more about preparing to stay focused and self-believing even when discussions reach a stage when you feel you have almost nothing sensible further to say.

In our experience, by recognising that there will be times when you are unable to add to what you have already said upon a subject, but by also knowing that you have prepared as thoroughly as you possibly could for your interview, **you will not lose your nerve**, and you will be able to continue and present yourself successfully.

With regard to *everything* **you say, or indeed have already submitted**, *prepare to justify* **your comments**.

To justify is to demonstrate the correctness, or actuality of an assertion.

So, for example, for every reference you make to any of your personal qualities, prepare to provide evidence; for every area of interest to which you refer, prepare to provide detailed examples.

For every viewpoint you have, prepare to explain it.

Keep asking yourself: *'How can I show them that I really mean what I say?'*

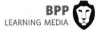

KEY POINTS

- You have been called to interview. You are a strong candidate.
- Believe in yourself. Prepare thoroughly.
- Always anticipate, and so prepare to respond to, the panel's relentless supplementary inquiry: *'Tell us exactly on what basis you have said that'.*
- If you cannot do that with real conviction, your statements will appear bland, empty, and lacking in substance.
- If you are able to do that, you will succeed!

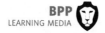

BPP
LEARNING MEDIA

Chapter 2

The medical school interview: the context

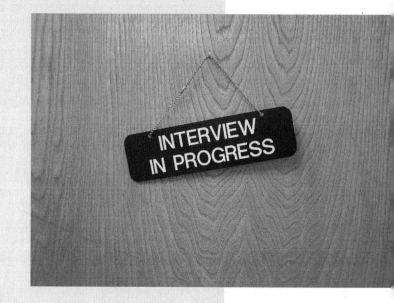

The medical school interview: the context

The process whereby students are selected to study Medicine is highly competitive. Most medical schools consider applications using a three-stage assessment process:

- The entrance examination.
- The candidate's UCAS application, which includes details of expected and achieved academic attainment, and their personal statement.
- The selection interview, when applicable.

Taking together the results of the entrance examination and the strength of the university application and personal statement, most medical schools then create the list of applicants they wish to interview.

What does it mean for you?

Well, to be called for interview is really good news. Your application to study medicine is on track. Alright, you are really not sure what will happen to you when you turn up, but it all seems very hopeful!

Yes, interviews are stressful experiences, there is no denying it. But with preparation and forethought you will be ready, and you have simply got to welcome this opportunity, make the very most of it, and *shine*!

Why do medical schools conduct interviews?

The important thing is – they are keen to see you, and talk to you in person. You look good on paper; they want to put a face to your application.

We shall look at the specific assessment criteria which universities apply when selecting medical students in Chapter 3 of this

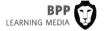

book. However, one of the first things to recognise from their perspective is that Medicine is an expensive course to run. It is also a fact that for every medical student who leaves the course, for whatever reason, there are significant financial implications (that is, costs!) to the university. So, one key reason they wish to meet you is for them to be able to come to an informed view as to whether or not you are likely to complete the course if you were offered a place.

Medical schools train the country's doctors of tomorrow. The expectation is, and this is enshrined in the Medical School Charter, that 'medical students undertake a degree in Medicine with the aim of becoming medical practitioners'. Now, it is the case that each year there are a small number of medical students who will obtain their degree but, for some reason, never practise Medicine at all. By meeting applicants face to face, this is another eventuality which medical schools are taking steps to avoid wherever possible.

A role that the medical school interview panel does NOT have as a priority is to assess your academic understanding and knowledge. The assessment of your academic core competencies for Medicine is largely done by considering your performance at formal examinations.

However, interview panels are extremely determined to get behind the words in your application submission and *form a view of what you are like as a person*; the interview is much more to do with assessing your suitability for the course and your personality.

Writing in general about the interview process in the *Sunday Times* in June 2011, the columnist, India Knight comments, '*There's a chasm between what someone's like on paper and what they're like in the flesh. Interviews fill the gaps. What you don't need is a bunch of charmless brainboxes whose only achievements are academic.*'

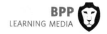

Behind all their inquiries, medical school interview panels are focusing upon the following key questions:

- *Are you passionate about studying Medicine?*
- *Do you have an understanding of what a career in Medicine entails and demands?*
- *If you were offered a place, would you complete the course?*
- *Will you fit in? How do you think you will contribute to life in this medical school? Are you suited to a medical career?*

What will your interview be like?

Usually, candidates are individually interviewed by the panel, although in recent years some medical schools have introduced group discussions as part of the assessment process.

There are usually three or four panel members, at least one being a senior doctor. Universities seek to balance the numbers of men and women on the panel, and try to obtain a mix of interviewers with different ethnic backgrounds, expertise and knowledge. Some panels have medical student representatives; some are keen to include a lay member of the public; some medical schools conduct mini-interviews where each candidate is seen by several small panels for a few minutes at a time.

Panels may use questions from a 'bank' formulated by the medical school. Other universities favour a mixed approach where questions are both pre-determined and also interviewer-led depending upon the candidate's responses and, importantly, submissions presented by the candidate within the application process, **especially their personal statement**.

More recently, applicants may be given a video to watch, an issue or problem to consider, or an article to read and then questioned on that material. Some medical schools are beginning to introduce problem-solving questions.

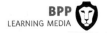

The interviews vary in length; most last between 15 and 40 minutes. Scoring systems vary too. Some schools ascribe numeric scores to the assessment criteria. Other medical schools arrive at an assessment of: offer/borderline/reject.

KEY POINT

- Your medical school interview is your key chance to convince the admissions tutors that you are an exceptional candidate and that they should offer you a place to study Medicine. Welcome it – and prepare to shine!

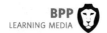

Chapter 3

What kind of students do medical schools want?

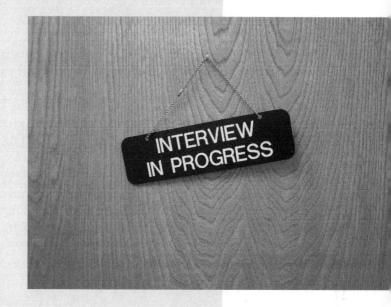

What kind of students do medical schools want?

Principles of selection and admission

The UK Council of Heads of Medical Schools, in consultation with the Department of Health and the British Medical Association has produced a statement setting out guiding principles underpinning the selection and admission of students to medical schools.

These principles detail that:

- **Selection for medical school implies selection for the medical profession.**

  A degree in Medicine in normal circumstances entitles the new graduate to be provisionally registered with the General Medical Council (GMC).

  Medical schools in the UK have a duty to ensure that the selection of students takes account of the qualities needed in a doctor as set out in the GMC's document '*Good Medical Practice*'.

  The practice of Medicine requires the highest standards of professional and personal conduct: always, the primary duty of care is to patients.

  It is vital that medical students understand and recognise this *from their first day*, and the implications of failing to do so.

  Experience suggests that some applicants will not be suited to a career in Medicine and it is in their best interest, and that of the public, that they are not admitted to medical school.

So, medical schools will be looking to select students who have academic ability AND a well rounded personality demonstrated by motivation and determination to study Medicine, wide-ranging interests, experience of team working – especially in health or social care settings, and leadership skills.

- **A high level of academic attainment will be expected.** And while understanding science is core to the understanding of Medicine, medical schools generally encourage diversity in subjects studied by candidates.
- **Candidates should demonstrate an understanding of what a career in Medicine involves.**

In line with these principles, university medical schools focus upon the importance of selecting students who best demonstrate:

- Factual understanding and *knowledge.*
- Interpersonal *skills*, especially communication skills within teams, the ability to remain calm under pressure, and to be able to demonstrate initiative and flexibility.
- Personal *attitudes* which reflect motivation towards medical study and ultimately appropriate behaviour as future doctors in their relationships with patients.

Students will also:

- Need to be determined individuals who are able to manage the stress which inevitably accompanies medical studies, and
- Contribute to the broad spectrum of university life. Those who do so are much more likely to gain a wider experience of working and communicating with people from different backgrounds.

In summary, medical schools aim to admit students who are most likely to become good doctors by gaining a solid grounding in core clinical knowledge and a thorough training in skills which

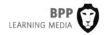

will equip them to become lifelong learners and effective team members.

The General Medical Council sets out definitions of 'good doctors' and the 'duties of a doctor':

Good doctors

Patients need good doctors. Good doctors make the care of their patients their first concern: they are competent, keep their knowledge and skills up to date, establish and maintain good relationships with patients and colleagues, are honest and trustworthy, and act with integrity.

The duties of a doctor

Patients must be able to trust doctors with their lives and wellbeing. To justify that trust, the profession has a duty to maintain a good standard of practice and care and to show respect for human life. In particular doctors must:

- Make the care of patients their first concern
- Treat every patient politely and considerately
- Respect patients' dignity and privacy
- Listen to patients and respect their views
- Give patients information in a way they can understand
- Respect the right of patients to be fully involved in decisions about care
- Keep their professional knowledge and skills up to date
- Recognise the limits of their professional competence
- Be honest and trustworthy
- Respect and protect confidential information
- Make sure that their personal beliefs do not prejudice their patients' care
- Act quickly to protect patients from risk if they have good reason to believe that they or a colleague may not be fit to practise
- Avoid abusing their position as a doctor; and

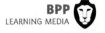

- Work with colleagues in the ways that best serve patients' interests.

In all these matters doctors must never discriminate unfairly against their patients or colleagues. And they must always be prepared to justify their actions to them.

Medical school interviews: assessment criteria

The principles set out above form the basis of the assessment criteria adopted by medical schools' interview panels.

Criterion 1: Evidence of ability to benefit from medical academic rigour

- While candidates' academic abilities are substantially assessed by reference to their achievements in formal examinations, prospective medical students need to demonstrate an understanding that **from the start of their studies they are responsible for their own learning.**

- A doctor is a person licensed to practise Medicine, which is the art and science of diagnosing and treating patients with symptoms and signs suggestive of disease. One of the main characteristics of a doctor is the ability to make decisions based upon a general assessment of the patient, taking into account both the important factual information and a recognition of the potential impact of influences that sometimes cannot be measured. Medical academic competency is not just the possession of abilities in scientific, objective reasoning. Taken to the extreme, those skills could lead to an approach towards caring for people which is indifferent and lacking in empathy.

In short, of course it is the case that good, effective medical practice depends upon sound *knowledge* and a relevant factual understanding. But it also requires the exercise

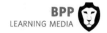

of clinical judgement, reflecting an astute *emotional intelligence*.

Criterion 2: Evidence of a rounded, maturing personality

The panel will be keen to explore **your**:

- Motivation and commitment to study Medicine; your awareness of medical issues, and why you believe you have what it takes to be a good doctor
- Experience of team working (especially in health or social service settings)
- Readiness to accept responsibility, and your awareness of your limitations
- Leadership skills
- Ability to express and defend **your** own views
- Strengths and weaknesses
- Determination, resolve and tenacity
- Lifestyle and interests outside studies
- Ways in which you relax

The interview also gives members of the panel a chance to gain some insight into those personal qualities so much associated with doctors – qualities such as kindness, compassion, empathy and curiosity. The panel will also reflect upon your general demeanour, attitude, and overall approach to life. They will be keen to assess whether you are always reliable, and whether you can handle the physical, mental and emotional strains you will experience, first as a medical student and then as a practising physician.

It is also very important for all candidates to understand that medical students' behaviour, including their behaviour outside the clinical environment and in their personal lives, may have an impact upon the assessment of their fitness to practise Medicine. Medical students' behaviour at all times must justify the trust the public places in the medical profession.

Criterion 3: Evidence of investment, or sacrifice, depicting a commitment to a future in Medicine

Consider the situation in which a Premier League Football Club is considering whether or not to offer a teenage boy with aspirations to be a professional footballer a position within the club's youth academy. You can be sure that in addition to their consideration of his football ability, the club's coaches will also be looking to see signs of a real commitment to a future career in the sport as demonstrated by, for example, his diet, and his attitude to drinking and smoking. In short, the club will be keen to see evidence of his personal investment in this career move. What is he especially keen to do? What is he prepared to give up?

The same applies to the consideration of medical school applications. So, the interview panel will be keen to find out how you spend your time outside the formal school curriculum. For example, do you try to keep abreast of medical developments as they are reported in leading scientific journals – such as *New Scientist, BMJ* – and in the national newspapers? Do you spend time at weekends supporting staff in a local hospice?

Criterion 4: Evidence of a compelling, interactive personality

A key implied question also underpins the panel's considerations on the day of the interview itself: does this candidate come over as *positive, self-believing, enthusiastic, fresh,* and *sincere* when talking about the prospect of studying Medicine and establishing a medical career?

KEY POINTS

- Selection for medical school implies selection for the medical profession.
- Medical schools want to select students who have more than just academic ability. They want to train good doctors for tomorrow.

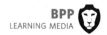

Chapter 4

Preparation for the medical school interview

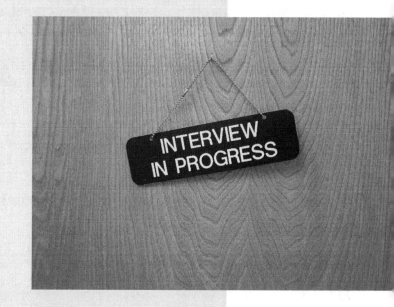

Chapter 4

Preparation for the medical school interview

The medical school interview is daunting, let there be no doubt about it.

During the course of their education, applicants have become used to being assessed by formal academic examinations, and especially, by such examinations in science subjects. So, many applicants will be very familiar with questions presented in the following form:

> *Describe what you would observe when anhydrous aluminium chloride is added to an excess of water. Write an equation for the reaction.*

In short, candidates for medical school are very experienced in satisfying examiners by referring to **facts**.

But medical school interviewers are interested in far more than facts. Indeed, if a candidate experienced an interview in which all the questions could be answered by factual recall, it could be said that the panel was not doing its job properly!

Before we go any further, let us set out three key definitions, and some basic principles underpinning the interview process.

Definitions

Fact: a thing that is known to have occurred, to exist or to be true.

Criterion: a principle or standard by which people judge something.

One's values: one's own consideration of what is important in life.

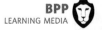

Some principles

- The medical school interview is a conversation between yourself and the panel. It is not an oral examination. However, it is also definitely NOT a chat!
- You have a mission: to convince the panel that you should be offered a place to study Medicine on their course.
- The panel have a mission: to offer places to those candidates who are assessed as best suited to study Medicine.
- The panel ask the questions; and there will be times when you are not quite sure what exactly you are being asked.
- It is for you to respond to those questions: and you may have to seek clarity upon what is being asked of you.

It is our experience that confident responses to the interviewers' questions are made when:

- *You make the interviewers' words mean what you want them to mean* (but without distorting their inquiry)
- For questions which explore your knowledge upon a topic or theme, *you have command of the relevant facts*
- For questions which explore your judgement, *you recourse to appropriate criteria,* and
- For questions which explore your own viewpoint and your approach to situations, *you feel comfortable about talking about yourself, and especially your personal values.*

We can illustrate this by imagining that someone who is a passionate tennis fan is asked the following questions:

Question
Who won the men's singles title at Wimbledon in 2011?

Fan's response
Novak Djokovic.

There is no doubt about this – it is a **fact!**

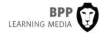

Chapter 4

Novak Djokovic defeated Rafael Nadal in the final.

Question

Who was the most successful tennis player in the men's game in 2011?

Fan's response

Well, again, the answer has to be Novak Djokovic.

Question

On what basis do you form that view?

Fan's response

Djokovic has won more major Grand Slam tournaments in the year than any other player in the men's game. In addition, the official world tennis ranking system, the ATP ranking, which takes into account players' results in all tournaments – and not just Grand Slam events – lifted him from Number 2 to Number 1 in the world in July, 2011.

In formulating responses to these two questions, the tennis fan has:

- Made the questioner's word *'successful'* mean what he wants it to mean. There could have been a conversation about what 'successful' meant in this context; the amount of money earned in the year, for instance, could have been one definition. Rather than seek clarification, the fan took the question 'head on' and responded in a confident way using their own definition.
- Referred to two key **criteria** in order to substantiate the appropriate use of the word 'successful'. These were:
  - The number of Grand Slam title wins in the given year, and;
  - The position on the ATP ranking system at a relevant point in time.

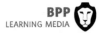

Question

Which player in men's tennis do you enjoy watching most?

Fan's response

For me it has to be Roger Federer.

Question

And why is that the case?

Fan's response

Well, to start with, I really admire his shots. His serve is not the fastest in the game, but his placement and use of different spins is amazing.

Then there is his fantastic movement around the court: it is almost like watching ballet.

The description as to why the fan *enjoyed* watching Federer most is not based on facts or criteria. They are such blunt, impersonal instruments when it comes to explaining any of our emotions.

The verbal content of this response reflects their own uniquely personal values; this fan appreciates accuracy more than power, and grace of movement rather than just strength and physical fitness.

Your medical school interview: why prepare?

Your ability to take a measured approach towards having a conversation and then applying this approach to the discussions you have with each member of the panel is fundamental to your chances of success.

In turn, members of the panel will be keen to see how you handle questions around matters of *fact*. Your responses to

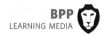

these questions will reflect your approach to the importance of accuracy and precision.

In addition, they will carefully consider the *criteria* to which you refer when explaining your judgements.

Panel members will also be looking to find out in what ways the passions and *values* you hold might affect the approaches you will bring to medical practice.

You need to equip yourself to be able to:

- Have a series of conversations with panel members on a wide range of themes.
- Justify *every* comment you make.
- Respond to *factual* questions **fluently**.
- Respond to questions which are designed to explore your judgement, your viewpoints and the approaches you might take, **carefully**.
- Welcome the panel's questions, even those which challenge you.
- Shine: be fresh, open, and passionate on the day, but always mindful that you are being assessed as a potential, future practising clinician, practice which begins the moment you take up your place as a medical student.

In short, you are preparing to be natural; not wooden and not obviously over rehearsed, but pleasantly confident and at ease with yourself.

How to prepare

The first consideration is that **you need time to prepare** and it is vital that you begin your efforts well in advance of any expected interview date. It is not at all uncommon for candidates to be invited to attend for interview on a date falling within one week of receiving their letter.

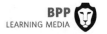

Ideally, we suggest that within about six months of your likely first medical school interview, you **start to assemble material**, including:

- Descriptions of yourself, according to yourself and others, such as your friends and teachers.
- Records, preferably in the form of diaries, of your work experience.
- Information about medical schools of your choice from the university websites.
- Articles about medical and health service issues which are published in national newspapers, and reviews of relevant television and radio programmes. These will prompt you to obtain:
  - Authoritative comments upon specific topics which you can access from scientific journals, either in libraries or via the internet.

Then, in the two months or so leading up to the day of the interview:

- **Select the specific topics** you are going to look at in detail by referring to the *Medical school interview: focused format* which is presented on page 29.
- For every topic, **imagine your interview to be made up of several separate pieces of question / answer discussions, each being based on up to three to four successive questions. Write down your imagined questions and then begin to frame your responses**.

Clearly, there is no guarantee at all that these imagined questions will actually form the basis of the panel's inquiries on the day. However, by adopting this approach, not only will you greatly add to your knowledge base, you will also be able to demonstrate that you truly do have a passion for the subject and a real understanding of what a career in Medicine involves **for you**.

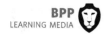

- **Keep these prepared responses in the form of a portfolio** which you can read in the days leading up to the interview.
- Then **practise what you might say on the day** with friends, teachers or members of your family.

Our experience suggests that you need to spend about 40 hours in dedicated preparation time in advance of your first interview.

Preparation for the interview: what to prepare

No student can possibly be expected to have detailed knowledge on every theme about which a member of the panel might ask at interview.

However, rightly or wrongly, fairly or unfairly, the panel will expect you to be able to converse sensibly upon any topic of their choosing.

Equally, there is no such thing as a 'standard' medical school interview.

However, we recommend that you used the *Focused format* because we believe it helps to ensure that all students preparing for their interviews, including graduate and mature students, will give careful consideration to those themes which, in our experience, are likely to come up one way or another.

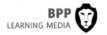

Medical school interview: focused format

Discussion / question themes:

1. Review of candidate's personal statement
2. Why do you want to study Medicine?
3. Why do you want to study Medicine at that specific university?
4. How do you know medicine is right for you, and that you are right for a medical career?
5. What are your strengths and weaknesses?
6. What are the biggest challenges facing the health service?
7. What is the most exciting medical development on the horizon?
8. Discussions about management; leadership; teamwork
9. Discussions about the importance of teaching.

We shall now look at how you might prepare for the panel's questions in each of these nine areas.

Preparation topic 1: The review of your personal statement

While it is possible that members of the panel have not been given sight of your personal statement, our advice is that you should thoroughly prepare to be able to handle questions upon its content. Indeed, **you have to welcome this!** After all, it is **your** statement; every word is important to **you**.

So:

- Make sure that you know the exact meaning of each *acronym* you have used. For example, that 'MRSA' is methicillin resistant staphylococcus aureus. And note; it is a kind of **bacterium**. In a recent 'mock' interview, one applicant explained that MRSA was a kind of virus. It is not a virus.

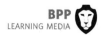

- Check out the exact meaning of any technical words or phrases you have used. For example, if you have used the word *'research'* be prepared to face questions upon its meaning, and be ready to provide an example.
  (Imagine the question: *'I see you are very interested in medical research. Can you give us an example of a piece of research which you found particularly interesting?'*)
- Make sure you can confidently explain any ambiguities or inconsistencies. For example, one applicant had written, *'I decided to take a gap year after my A level examinations'* and yet later in his personal statement he wrote, *'I studied Biology at university for six weeks before leaving that course and going to Australia'*. Careful preparation for his interview enabled that candidate to anticipate the awkward questions from the panel, and to provide a sincere apology for accidentally presenting ambiguous information.
  Equally, check to see, for example, which examples of your strengths you refer to in your personal statement. To respond to an interview question by describing something quite different would certainly raise some eyebrows!
- If you have said that you enjoy reading certain kinds of articles or books, **be ready with your examples.** So, as part of your preparation, it would be extremely valuable to write out a short summary (say 100 words) of any book or article to which you have specifically referred in your personal statement.
- Indeed, **you must prepare to be able to speak fluently and enthusiastically about any topic or theme that you raise, either in your personal statement or anywhere else in your application, or during the interview itself.** To speak tentatively about topics which you introduce gives a very bleak impression indeed.

Let us look at this principle in more detail. For illustrative purposes, suppose you are preparing for a medical school interview having submitted your personal statement in which you had stated the following:

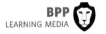

'I really enjoy taking part in our school journal club. Every month one of us gives a presentation on interesting recent issues: when my turn came, I spoke about issues relating to 'abortion' and 'assisted suicide'.

By referring to specific medical topics, the panel members will infer that you are encouraging questions upon these themes.

And, so long as you have prepared carefully, that could turn out to be very much to your advantage.

However, take note: having invited discussions upon these subjects by referring specifically to them in your personal statement, you must anticipate that the interviewers may take the opportunity to ask you *anything* they wish to with regard to these two health topics.

Framing your responses to imagined questions upon these themes provides an excellent opportunity for you to consider the importance of **facts**, of **criteria** by which you justify your comments, and of **your own personal values** (within a **medical ethics** framework) in equipping you to be able to discuss these topics with confidence. So, let us look at the first topic: namely, issues relating to 'abortion'. In this regard, consideration of the basic principles of medical ethics will be extremely helpful towards preparing your responses to questions from the panel.

Principles of medical ethics

The medical profession has historically subscribed to a core set of ethical principles which aim to reflect the needs of patients. Doctors are required to recognise their responsibility to patients first and foremost, as well as to the wider society, to other health professionals, and to themselves.

Ethical principles are NOT laws, but they are standards of professional conduct.

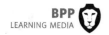

The principles provide a valuable framework for the consideration of complex moral health issues. In preparing for your interview, you will find the following principles deserve particular attention.

These are the principles of:

1. Beneficience: A doctor should act in the best interest of the patient.

2. Non-maleficience: As a priority, a doctor should do no harm.

3. Autonomy: The patient has the right to refuse, or to choose, their treatment.

4. Justice: Professional actions carried out by doctors should also take regard of the impact such actions have on the wider society. Summed up, it reads: 'Fairness for all'.

It is this principle which should apply in consideration of:

- The distribution of scarce resources
- Decisions around 'who gets what' treatment
- The impact of medical decisions upon healthcare professionals themselves, such as those relating to terminations of pregnancy, or to terminal care.

As before, let us imagine how the questioning might proceed.

Imagined question 1

'I see you looked at issues relating to abortion in your presentation to the journal club. Which issues did you consider?'

This is a simple question seeking a factual description of the content of your presentation. You must be prepared for this! It might be that you had accessed the website *NHS Choices* and used the information to enable you to speak about the legal position, or about the difficulties people have in coming to their decision to terminate a pregnancy. Or perhaps you had seen the clutch of articles in several scientific journal websites (such as *Nature* and the *New England Journal of Medicine*) in January 2011, in which the results of a study looking at the potential impact abortions had upon women's mental health were described.

Whichever specific issues you had touched upon at the journal club, it is vital that you are able to give a fluent, factual response to this inquiry.

Imagined question 2

'Why did you decide to look at issues relating to abortion?'

Here the interviewer is seeking to learn of the criteria by which you judged that the consideration of this topic would be valuable for yourself and for the students attending your presentation. If, for example, you responded by saying that you really hadn't known what to speak about, and that you had asked your tutor for advice and it was at his suggestion that you had looked at the subject of abortion, then the panel may well form a bleak impression of your enthusiasm and passion for speaking at the journal club.

However, if you were to explain that you had been struck by the number of articles commenting upon mental health and abortion (implying that there was considerable interest in this topic amongst health professionals), AND that you had realised that by focusing upon this subject you could then prompt a useful discussion about medical ethics amongst the students attending your presentation, then you would be clearly showing the panel that you had given careful thought as to how you might use your presentation to its best effect.

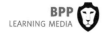

Imagined question 3

> *'I see you looked at issues relating to abortion when you spoke to the journal club. Do you think it is right for women to obtain abortion on demand?'*

What a stark, direct, personal question. Look at how extreme some of the language is – the use of the words *'right'* and *'demand'*. And you can have no idea as to the views of the interviewer on this matter. Certainly, this is no time to take a guess at where you believe they stand and then form a response which you hope will please them.

Yes, there is a great deal of statistical information available; for example, the numbers of terminations carried out each year, how many are conducted for different age groups of pregnant women, how many at different gestational ages of the foetus.

But it is clear that any command you have of this kind of factual information cannot possibly provide the basis of your response to this question. Neither are there criteria to which you can turn.

Your response to this question will be framed by your **values, the qualities you believe are important in life**. The question calls for **you** to tell the panel **about you**; they are not concerned to learn how others see this particular issue at all!

Some members of the panel will be very experienced in ruffling candidates; indeed, some enjoy doing it. They know that many students reflect the approach taken by the interviewer in terms of conversational style and general demeanour, the length of sentences, the kinds of words and expressions used, and so on. So, in response to a short, sharp question, (like this one!) many students instinctively come back with an equally short, sharp reply. In mirroring the interviewer, they reflect the brevity and urgency of the question.

But you can be sure that if you were to reply to the question with the ultimate brevity – be it by a **'yes'** or a **'no'** answer to this question – the interviewer would then follow it up with the inquiry *'and why do you hold that view?'*, so keeping the pressure right on!

In situations like this, it is vital for you to understand that **the panel will not be impressed by a glib, succinct reply.** You must develop your response carefully, even if you believe by so doing you are causing the interviewer to be exasperated. So, take a deep breath before rushing into making any comments.

Forming your response

If you really are jarred by the tone adopted by the interviewer, then make the words of the question, *'Do you think it is right for women to obtain abortion on demand?'* mean what **you** want them to mean, but still in keeping with the line of inquiry.

It is very clear that the question aims to find out about your own views with regard to abortions. So equip yourself to respond to the somewhat more measured question, *'Where do you stand with regard to abortions: are you for or against them?'*

People generally take one of three main stances on abortion: pro-abortion, anti-abortion, and the middle ground that abortion is acceptable in some circumstances, such as in the event of rape, or the exploitation of women.

To help you form a careful measured view as to where you stand, the medical ethical principles provide a valuable framework around which the issues can be considered.

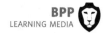

Ethical arguments used to support abortion

Autonomy: Some take the view that abortion represents a woman's right to exercise control over her own body.

(However, this does raise the questions: Is not the foetus a person with their own rights, too? Are the rights of the foetus less important than for someone who has already been born?)

Beneficience: Abortions will always be sought by women who are desperate and it is better for society to have safe termination services.

Justice: It is argued that in the interests of society, there should be as few unwanted children in the world as possible.

Arguments used against abortion

Non-maleficience: Many who stand against abortion do so because of their view that abortion challenges the sanctity of human life; they see abortion as a form of murder. They also argue that the procedure trivialises the potential psychological effects of abortions upon women and health professionals.

Justice: Acceptance of abortion is seen by some to encourage irresponsible attitudes to contraception.

More widely, the view is held that by permitting abortions, the respect society feels for other vulnerable humans is diminished. An impression is created that the only so called 'valuable' people are those who conform to a notion of normality. Some fear that ultimately, this could potentially lead to the acceptance of involuntary euthanasia.

So, use your preparation time to consider carefully where you stand on the issues.

Perhaps you are someone who is genuinely not particularly troubled by the ethical dilemmas relating to the termination of pregnancy. If that is the case, then you need to be very careful when you explain this to the panel. In our recent mock interviews, one student described that he would have *'no problems with carrying out abortions'*, and another explained that she had *'no sympathy at all for women who requested terminations of pregnancy'*. Of course, as soon as they had made these statements, their descriptions of themselves as empathic, caring and compassionate human beings all sounded a bit hollow!

On the other hand, if you are concerned about aspects of the procedure, you must anticipate possible further questions exploring how your views might affect your interactions with patients.

Imagined question 4

'Do you think there might be occasions when your views might affect the way you relate to patients who seek abortions?'

In asking this question, the interviewer is actually seeking to find out if it is possible that you might allow your views on the issues to get in the way of doing what is right for the patient.

So reflect carefully:

* Are you someone who will use the privilege of their position as a medical student, or as a doctor, to try to persuade patients to act in ways which **you** think are right for them?

The General Medical Council provides clear guidance on matters like this, recognising that personal beliefs and values, and cultural and religious practices are central to the lives of doctors and

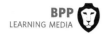

patients: and that all doctors have personal beliefs which affect their day-to-day practice.

Importantly, the guidance further states:

> *'But doctors must not impose their beliefs on patients or pressure patients to justify their beliefs. If carrying out a particular procedure or giving advice about it conflicts with your religious or moral beliefs, and this conflict might affect the treatment or advice you provide, you must explain this to the patient and tell them they have the right to see another doctor.'*

You should also understand that, according to the law, a doctor can be sued for damages if, because of a failure to refer, a delay is caused which results in the woman being unable to obtain a termination.

- Are you someone who has such strong views that you would not wish to take part in abortion procedures?

The Abortion Act of 1967 exempts doctors, and indeed any healthcare professional, from an obligation to participate in abortion.

> *'No person shall be under any duty to participate in the treatment authorised in the Abortion Act to which he has a conscientious objection.'*

Advice provided by the British Medical Association (See Glossary) is that its members, which include medical students, should always act within the law and according to their own conscience.

Now let us look at the second topic to which you refer in your personal statement, namely issues relating to assisted suicide.

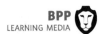

Imagined question 1

'With regard to your presentation to the journal club, what exactly is the current legal position on assisted suicide?'

On the face of it, this is a simple question requiring a factual answer. However, in your response, you will need to explain that different countries have different legal positions. In the United Kingdom, while attempting to commit suicide is not itself a criminal act, assisted suicide is illegal under the terms of the Suicide Act of 1961 and is punishable by up to 14 years' imprisonment.

However, in the Netherlands, euthanasia is legalised under certain very specific circumstances, and in Switzerland, a person can avoid conviction for assisted suicide if they were able to prove the patient knew what they were doing, had capacity to make the decision and had requested to die on several occasions.

Imagined question 2

'Why do you think this subject has received so much media attention recently?'

In considering the subject before your presentation to the journal club, you may well have read of:

- Instances of distinguished people travelling to the Dignitas clinic in Switzerland, and there being helped to commit suicide; for example, the great musical conductor Edward Downes, in July, 2009.
- The television coverage of Sir Terry Pratchett accompanying a man who suffered from motor neurone disease to the Dignitas clinic. The death of this patient was the first time suicide had been broadcast on terrestrial television, sparking a fierce debate.
- Efforts made by Debbie Purdy, a woman suffering from a terminal illness who launched a two-day judicial review

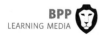 BPP
LEARNING MEDIA

at London's High Court in an effort to force the Crown Prosecution Service to spell out exactly what actions would lead a friend or relative open to being charged with aiding or abetting her suicide. Subsequently, in 2010, guidelines for prosecutors in cases of assisted suicide were established. (See 'Euthanasia' in the Glossary section of this book).

Clearly, many newspaper articles and television programmes have commented upon the actions taken by high profile people at the end of their own, or someone else's life, and the passionate efforts by others to obtain clarity around the law. These articles and programmes have generated much debate and considerable media attention to issues around 'assisted suicide' in recent years.

Imagined question 3

'And why did the subject of 'assisted suicide' interest you so much?

Now be careful. It may indeed be that you are someone who wants to change the world, and that you have developed a determination to work with others towards achieving a change in the law. However, if the panel sense this, you can be sure that they will try to find out just how much your passion in this field might affect the way you relate to patients, and work with colleagues.

You will be less likely to get into difficulties if you explain that you felt that the consideration of the ethical issues relating to abortion and assisted suicide, together, provided a real learning opportunity for yourself and your student colleagues. It may also have been that you had been inspired by the book written about Matt Hampson, the rugby player who had been paralysed following the collapse of a scrum in 2006. In a review article in the *Telegraph Online* in August 2011, far from contemplating means by which he might seek to end his life, he is quoted as being keen to 'get out and show that there are people in wheelchairs with pipes hanging from their neck living a life.'

So, reflect carefully and honestly upon the values you hold dear. Consider carefully their implications upon your possible conduct, firstly as a medical student, and then as a practising doctor.

Prepare to speak comfortably and with confident self-belief about your values and perspectives.

Preparation topic 2: Why do you want to study Medicine?

It is almost certain that you will be asked to explain why it is that, out of all academic courses on offer, you are so very keen to study Medicine. It is vital for you to use the time leading up to your interview to prepare your response to this question with passion, enthusiasm and conviction.

What is Medicine?

To study Medicine at university is to learn about the science of the human body in health and disease, and then to apply that knowledge when caring for patients and working alongside colleagues. To practise Medicine is to combine effective communication with practical skills.

Every medical student has their own story as to how and why they came to make that academic – and career – choice.

At one recent medical school open day, two junior doctors gave a talk in which they looked back at how they had been inspired to study Medicine.

In their presentation, they touched upon the following themes.

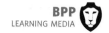

- The sheer breadth of the subject. Yes, subjects such as Biology and Chemistry are fundamental to gaining an understanding of Medicine, but there are also important connections to Physics, Statistics, Social Sciences and Politics.

  The career choices open to new graduates are enormous: the clinical care of people from cradle to grave, preventative medicine and public health, research, teaching, and, increasingly, management.

- Medical practice is focused on helping people. Medicine is not metaphysics; it is an applied discipline.

  To embark upon a medical career is to commit a professional lifetime in trying to improve the health and welfare of people from all kinds of backgrounds suffering from many different illnesses and disabilities.

  Yes, the public respect, admire and appreciate doctors as professionals. But that serves as a reminder that there is no place for arrogance or self-satisfaction. To practise Medicine is a privilege, and a truly humbling experience.

- The fascination is never ending, be it today's complex diagnostic case, causing concern to the patient and their loved ones alike, or the identification of genetic patterns which in the future may powerfully influence ethical and political debates.

You also need to prepare to respond to challenging questions from the panel on this subject, such as:

Imagined question 1

'What will you do if you don't receive any offers this year to study Medicine?'

There are many successful doctors in practice today who failed to obtain a place in their first round of applications. Indeed, it

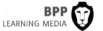

is often the case that those who entered medical studies after an early disappointment ultimately become the most successful. If you are truly determined, failure to be selected will only serve to spur you on.

Imagined question 2

'Will you really be able to cope with the emotional side of it all?'

How do you know that you will be able to handle the 'messy' aspects of medical study? Have you encountered this kind of challenge before? What did you learn from the experience?

There are indeed stories of students leaving the course after their first practical session of anatomic dissection, or fainting at the start of experiments in which the physiology of cerebral function is examined in decerebrate cats!

And then you go on to meet real patients with real diseases!

When you describe why you are so passionately keen to study Medicine at the interview, you must do it in your own words.

However, you can be sure that the panel members will be looking to see evidence of **passion** and careful **reflection** in your comments.

Preparation topic 3: Why do you want to study Medicine at that specific university?

Again, you will almost certainly be asked this question during your interview, and it is very important that you are able to explain the reasons for your choice.

Each medical school has their own selection process, so make sure you visit their website in order to obtain the necessary details.

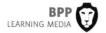

Chapter 4

University 'Open Days' are extremely valuable in helping you to decide where you wish to study so it is vital that you visit the medical school in advance of your interview.

As part of your preparation, reflect upon the following:

- Do you want to remain near home during your medical studies?

- Would you prefer to study at a campus or a city-based medical school?

- Do you feel comfortable in the locality in which the medical school is set?

    By far the majority of doctors in the UK take up their substantive posts in the vicinity of the medical school at which they trained. So it is important that you consider the recreational and cultural attractions of the area.

- Will you enjoy their educational approaches?

    These do vary. During the last ten years or so, medical education has changed considerably with many medical schools reorganising their courses. The emphasis now is not so much directed towards students gaining the knowledge required to undertake the duties of a doctor; it is about them obtaining essential knowledge together with a thorough training in lifelong learning skills.

    Some courses are based very largely on problem-based learning, an approach in which teaching is student-centred and directed, with the focus placed on the consideration of case studies or scenarios. Students present their findings in the context of achieving defined educational objectives.

    Some universities offer the opportunity for students to gain experience in full body anatomic dissection; others use computer generated imagery for these sessions.

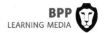

- When will you begin to interact with patients?

  Some medical schools, but by no means all, are keen to ensure that students meet patients very early in their course.

- Are you keen to take advantage of additional academic opportunities?

  Some medical schools include the BMedSci degree, so that after five years their students emerge with two degrees. Many provide the chance to spend some time studying abroad.

Within the interview, you might also be asked:

- Which other medical schools have you applied to?
- Have you attended, or are you expecting to attend, interviews at other universities?
- Are there any aspects of our course which put you off in some way?

These questions may seem to be unfair and they make you feel uncomfortable. However, when responding, it is vital that you tell the truth. Remember: there are many students who complete their medical studies at a university which was not their first choice.

Preparation topic 4: Confirming that Medicine is right for you and that you are right for Medicine

It is vital that you are able to demonstrate to the interview panel that you have a good understanding of what medical studies, and then a future medical career, entail.

It is a long degree course; for most students it will be five years before they start earning. Most of your friends going to university will gain their degree two years earlier than you.

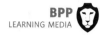

The course demands a considerable study effort; it is not like Mathematics, for example, where the naturally talented really do have a tangible advantage.

Then there is the stress and emotional strains that caring for patients brings, particularly dealing with people who are very ill, some of them dying. Will you be able break bad news to people?

You really will need to convince the panel that you are able to engage appropriately with distressed and disabled people and that you are able to draw near in support of them.

> **NOTE:**
> There is no place for arrogance or self-satisfaction in a medical career. Setting a course on becoming a doctor is a humbling experience. It is indeed a 'way of life'.

And it is probably wise that you do NOT explain in detail why you are *certain* that that you want to be, say, a general practitioner. By all means indicate where your longer term career interests might presently lie. But anyone with a real commitment to 'lifelong learning' must recognise that their views might change in the light of their experiences as their medical training progresses.

Your work experience

It is vital that you review your work experience when preparing for inquiries around these themes.

Medical schools expect applicants to benefit from a range of relevant work experience in two ways.

- To obtain insights into the way healthcare professionals carry out their work. (That is, helping you to find out if Medicine is right for you.)

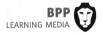

The panel will be especially interested to hear if you have been able to talk directly with different doctors about their careers and the issues facing them in the 21st century.

- To help you develop the relevant attributes and personal qualities which will enable you to become a good doctor. (That is, to further enable you to become right for Medicine.)

  Important amongst these are your developing sense of responsibility, reliability and service; increasing your self-awareness; strengthening your determination and ability to handle difficulties; and building up your confidence both as a team member and, when necessary, your ability to work independently.

  Your work experience also provides excellent opportunities for you to appreciate the importance of, and further develop your own, communication skills.

Communication skills

Medical schools place great emphasis upon the importance of effective communication skills when selecting medical students. From very early in your course you will be expected to communicate clearly and sensitively with patients and their relatives, as well as with colleagues from professional groups.

Hopefully, your work experience will increase your understanding of the value of:

- Listening, and especially acknowledging the comments of someone talking to you.
- Taking time to explain at the outset of a conversation the topics which are going to be covered.
- Focusing on *positive* messages, and providing encouragement.
- Presenting questions in a sincere, open way, so as to welcome discussion rather than seek to obtain merely 'yes' or 'no' responses.

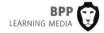

- Handling telephone conversations with great care. Whenever information is imparted without a formal record being retained, the need for clarity and understanding becomes even more paramount.
- Preparation before very significant discussions, such as the breaking of bad news to patients. For example, the importance of considering the setting in which to present such information.
- Considering the issue of confidentiality. It is perfectly understandable that a close family member should ask questions about the outlook for a loved one who is very ill. However, it is vital that the patient's views are sought in advance, and any request for confidentiality respected.
- Different forms of communication, including spoken, written, and electronic methods. You might also gain insights into how best to communicate with vulnerable people, including those suffering from disabilities such as deafness and blindness, and with individuals who cannot speak English, or who come from a very different cultural background.
- **Learning** from your experiences: as part of your preparation, a very good discipline is to keep a diary so that you can reflect upon what you have achieved and what you have learned, especially perhaps when things did not go exactly according to plan!

Questions you might be asked relating to your work experience

- *'What challenged you most during your work experience?'*
  'Did this experience indicate that perhaps you were not cut out for medicine?'
- *'What new insights did you obtain?'*
- *'Did your work experience lead to you changing your mind or reviewing your situation?'*
- *'What new skills did you obtain?'*
- *'Describe one event that made a strong positive impression upon you.'*
- *'Describe one event that jarred you.'*

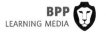

- *'Describe one situation – which you observed or in which you played some part – where poor communication affected events.'* *'What did you learn from that?'*

Preparation topic 5: What are your strengths and weaknesses?

This question should have a health warning attached to it: the inquiry invites calamity. For any of us, the invitation to talk about our strengths provides the opportunity for us to take it all too far; the response can so easily drift towards an expression of arrogant pride.

And to ask about our weaknesses in an interview setting is as challenging as it gets. Who wants to admit to any? And yet we all have weaknesses, even the members of the panel.

So, prepare to get through this question as carefully as possible. Dismiss the temptation to be arrogant and make sure that your descriptions of any weaknesses are not the cause of your downfall.

And imagine the follow up questions:

- *'Who benefits from your strengths?'*
  Hopefully, you will be able to describe how your strengths add to the contributions you make to the teams in which you play a part.

  And make sure you check your personal statement, and stay consistent. Any strengths to which you refer in your personal statement must be listed again. Now is not the time to change things; it will look to be contrived.

  Be ready to evidence your strengths: you will need examples. But it must not be an ego trip; so don't start every sentence with 'I'.

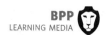
BPP
LEARNING MEDIA

- *'Who is affected by your weaknesses?'*
  Now is not the time to open up to your biggest flaws –
  or worse, any weakness which you feel to be potentially
  destructive.

  For example, to admit to being unreliable in a way that
  repeatedly hinders your performance within a team, is
  tantamount to disqualifying yourself from selection to
  medical school.

  Not to raise such aspects of your personality in response
  to this question from the panel is, of course, prudent: but
  if you really are affected in a way such as this perhaps you
  should reflect – are you really right for Medicine?

  So, prepare to admit to some 'safe' weaknesses. And these
  will not be personality qualities (such as, for example, 'I
  know I lack empathy at times'), because none of us can
  really change our personality.

  Having a weakness in computing skills seems a fair example;
  it should not affect your performance within a team too
  much, and it is in an area you can do something about.

  **And this brings us to an important principle: your
  weaknesses are your development areas, and we all have
  some of them! They're all about 'work in progress'.**

  Some weaknesses may be irritations associated with strengths.
  For example, if you believe one of your strengths is attention
  to accuracy and detail, others might at times perceive you
  to be pedantic, someone who seems to block progress or
  at least slow things down seemingly for the sake of it. You
  could lessen the impact of that perception by recognising
  it, and requesting the opportunity to express your views
  upon a situation as early as possible.

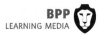

But do not sound glib, or slick, by saying that someone's weaknesses can often be the same as their strengths. You will be asked to evidence that, and you will run into difficulties.

NOTE:
Practise potential discussions with friends. Feel comfortable about your admitted weaknesses.

Be satisfied, but not smug, about your strengths.

You might be asked other questions on this subject, such as:
- **What would you change about yourself?**
- **If we were to ask one of your friends to describe what your biggest strengths and weaknesses are, what would they say?**
- **What is your most significant fault?**

Preparation topic 6: What are the biggest challenges facing the health service?

When considering how you would respond to this question, it is important to understand that there is no right answer. In addition, we suggest that you prepare to be able to discuss more than one topic area: at the end of a conversation from which you emerge with a sense of relief thinking that it is over, it is just so easy for an interviewer to then ask 'and are there are any other challenges which the health service is facing?'

Whatever your selection, the panel will be keen to explore:

- Your factual understanding of the subject
- Your justification of the choice of topic, and
- Your own individual personal perspectives, such as where you stand on related ethical issues, or why it is that you have become so interested in this area.

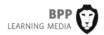

For illustrative purposes, we will look at three areas of challenge:

- The rising demand for healthcare from the elderly population.
- The continuing threat presented by infectious diseases.
- Challenges relating to London hosting the Olympic Games in 2012.

For each of these topic areas we will focus upon:

a. **Assembling a factual understanding**
   We suggest that, for three to six months before your interview, you keep abreast of ALL health-related articles published in, say, two of the country's leading national daily newspapers.

   And in order to gain a more detailed understanding of the specific topics which will form the basis of your focused preparation, we suggest you access relevant authoritative publications, many of which are readily available via the internet.

b. **The justification of your selection of this topic** as an important challenge.

c. **Why YOU find this topic interesting**: your personal perspective.

So, let us begin by looking at how you might prepare to respond to questions from the panel relating to the challenge posed by the rising demand for healthcare from the elderly population.

Assembling a factual understanding: material from national newspapers
During your weeks of preparation, you may have come across articles such as *Numbers of elderly people in hospital surge* by Rebecca Smith, the *Telegraph Online*, October 28th, 2010.

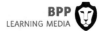

In this piece, it is described that the number of old people being treated in hospitals has risen by almost two-thirds in the last decade.

Assembling a factual understanding: authoritative sources via the internet

The website www.radcliffe-oxford.com is a gateway providing access to several excellent articles which consider health issues affecting the elderly. For example, you will be able to read Chapter 8 of Donaldson's *Essential Public Health*, entitled *Health in Later Life*, in which the authors explain the dramatic increase in the average length of life of men and women over the last hundred years, as well as describing how diseases and disabilities impact upon the quality of life of so many old people. They comment that very old people rarely suffer from a single disease and rely for care upon health professionals from many disciplines – such as medicine, nursing, physiotherapy.

In 2001, the Department of Health published *A National Service Framework for Older People*, a document which set out national standards for healthcare of older people. In 2006, the Department published *A New Ambition for Old Age* which sets out the next steps in implementing that original *National Service Framework*.

These important statements touch upon the need to change society's attitudes towards older people so that they become more valued and respected. The publications also highlight the need for more services for old people suffering strokes, falls, and chronic conditions, such as diabetes.

Both of these Department of Health publications are accessible via the internet.

The justification of your selection of this topic

If, in your reading of all health-related articles in the national press you had come across the piece in the *Daily Telegraph* on

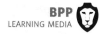

September 1st, 2011, entitled *Cut hospitals and consultants, says ex-NHS chief* by Martin Beckford, you would have seen reference to the following statement made by Lord Crisp, Chief Executive of the NHS from 2000 to 2006: '*…the main problem facing the health service was the growth in long-term conditions, such as diabetes, and the increasing number of elderly people.*'

You may also have seen comments made by Lord Darzi presented in the *Telegraph Online* on June 7th, 2011, in which he describes '*addressing rising demands from an ageing population*' as one of his four challenges for the health service. (Lord Darzi is Professor of Surgery at the Institute of Cancer Research, and in 2009 was appointed the United Kingdom's Global Ambassador for Health and Life Sciences.)

Coming from two experts so steeped in experience, the shared observation of these two Lords on what comprises a major challenge for the health service is certain to be worthy of careful consideration.

Why you find this topic so interesting?
Just consider the following imagined question.

'*OK. So you say that it was the comments of Lord Crisp and Lord Darzi that convinced you that caring for elderly people is a major challenge to the health service. But what do you think?*'

Here, the interviewer is trying to get behind, perhaps even disrupt, that scholarly, academic approach upon which you have based your responses to the questions on this subject so far. And what on earth does he mean by asking, '*what do you think*'?

Now, you could enter into a laboured discussion in which you seek to further clarify the specifics of that question. But you can rest assured, that conversation will lead you out of your comfort zone. Why not be brave and make the words of the question mean what you want them to mean, and treat it as an

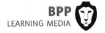

opportunity to talk about what had really interested you as you explored the subject.

For example, the statistician in you might have been fascinated by the fact that not only are the numbers of elderly increasing over the next several years, but the rates at which some diseases occur in the elderly population are also increasing – comprising a double, even 'exponential', challenge to the health service.

Or it may be that you had gained some insight into the health problems suffered by old people during your work experience, and this encouraged you to read more widely around the subject.

In whatever way you do respond to this question, it is vital that you demonstrate real enthusiasm for the subject.

Now let us consider how you might look at the challenge posed by some infectious diseases.

Assembling a factual understanding: material from national newspapers

In preparing for your interview, you may have come across articles in the national press such as:

- *200,000 would die and public order could breakdown in flu pandemic* by Martin Beckford, Health Correspondent for the *Telegraph* writing on March 23rd 2011. In this piece the journalist states that an '*outbreak of a new influenza pandemic is one of the greatest threats facing the UK.*'
- *London – the TB capital of Europe* by Stephen Adams, Medical Correspondent for the *Telegraph* writing on December 17th, 2010. It is stated within this article that more than 9,000 cases of TB are diagnosed annually in the UK, and that some doctors suggest that these numbers underestimate the problem by almost a third.
- *More than 330 measles cases in just four months* also written by Martin Beckford, in the *Telegraph* on May 27th, 2011. The

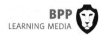

writer describes that this number represents a ten-fold rise compared to the same period in the previous year.

Assembling a factual understanding: authoritative sources via the internet

- The Department of Health *UK Influenza Pandemic Preparedness Strategy*, which states that *'Pandemic influenza is one of the most severe natural challenges likely to affect the UK.'*
- The National Electronic Library for Medicine, which on December 20th, 2010, provided a summary of the paper in *The Lancet* from which the *Telegraph Online* obtained statistics about tuberculosis in London.
- The website www.bmj.com on June 15th, 2011, had a piece entitled *Measles outbreak in Europe* by Simon Cottrell and Richard John Roberts, who write, *'Current outbreaks of measles in Europe are a reminder of the important risks of death and serious morbidity associated with measles.'*

By studying these several articles, you will be able to gain an excellent factual understanding of the subject.

The justification of your selected topic

Clearly, the numbers of cases in themselves provide some justification for your selection of this topic. However, these conditions present challenges which extend so much more widely than simply the distress they cause to the suffering patients. For example, the *UK Influenza Preparedness Strategy* document has sections entitled *The impact of school closure on an influenza pandemic*, and *The impact of mass gatherings on an influenza pandemic*. Within that document there is also a section detailing an attempt to estimate the potential impact of such a pandemic upon the UK economy. The authors provide illustrative figures based upon an assumption of illness-related absence from work affecting 50% of employees for roughly one and a half weeks per person. In this scenario, they estimate the costs of such a pandemic to the nation might amount to £28 billion.

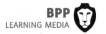

With regard to the challenge associated with tuberculosis, Britain is currently the only Western European country with rising rates of the disease, and commentators have called for serious long term political and financial commitment to control the impact of the disease. And measles, which had been thought to have been almost eradicated, is an extremely infectious and potentially dangerous disease: very many cases require to be hospitalised. The challenge associated with the rise in the numbers of cases of measles relates importantly to the need to address the failure of an immunisation programme, with around 85% of cases having been unvaccinated.

Why you find this topic so interesting?
The interviewer may ask: *'What was it that really caught your attention with regard to this particular threat?'*

Now, it may have been that your reading around the issues created in you a sense of awe at the ability of bacteria and viruses to adapt and survive the man-made efforts to curb their impact, such as via the use of antibiotics and immunisation programmes.

Or you may have become interested in the role played by social factors in explaining the increase in numbers of cases of some infectious diseases. For example, it is considered that conditions associated with poverty – run-down housing, poor ventilation, and overcrowding – in which some people live in London may be an important factor in their developing tuberculosis.

Finally in this section, let us look at how you might prepare to take questions from the panel about the challenges which accompany London hosting the Olympic Games in 2012.

When it was announced, in July 2005, that the Olympic Games would be coming to London in 2012, the International Olympic Committee explained that their decision had recognised the city's ambitious plans which promised a health promoting legacy

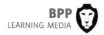

aimed at involving more of the country's young people in sport and physical exercise.

In addition, hosting the Games provides a once in a lifetime opportunity for London, and indeed the country as a whole, to demonstrate to the world the quality of the nation's health services, and health promotion programmes.

It is estimated that over the course of the late summer of 2012

- Around 17,000 athletes and officials are expected to stay in the Olympic village, and
- Around 9 million ticket holders will be supporting the competitions at approximately 200 sporting venues in and around the capital.

However, it is also recognised that the flow of very large numbers of young people into the city from all over the world carries an accompanying increased threat to the health of those participating in, and those supporting, the events.

Assembling a factual understanding: material from national newspapers

With regard to the health threat, the piece by James Meikle in the *Guardian* on July 14th, 2011, entitled *NHS: Shakeup of public health body delayed until after Olympics*, comments upon the importance of careful planning for the emergency response to potential serious incidents occurring at the Games, such as food poisoning or a biochemical terrorist act.

There are also articles which comment upon the prospects of gaining the health legacy in the run up and aftermath of the Games, such as that written in the *Telegraph* on May 20th, 2010, headed *No evidence that 2012 Olympics will improve health or wealth*. This presented the opinions of public health specialists at Glasgow University who had looked at 54 studies assessing the health impact of major multi-sport events since 1978. They

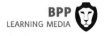

concluded that health benefits from the 2012 Olympic Games could not be expected to occur automatically.

Assembling a factual understanding: authoritative pieces available via the internet

Again, to help broaden your understanding of the threats to health presented by the Olympic Games, there are several valuable articles published on the internet by the Health Protection Agency (HPA). For example, in their publication *Olympics and Paralympics 2012: HPA Concept of Operations*, there is detailed analysis of the potential increased risks of diseases associated with the influx of large numbers of international visitors coming together at mass gatherings and in restricted space; there are sections looking at the need for vigilance with regard to food safety, water safety and air quality.

NHS London, the Strategic Health Authority which has lead responsibility for promoting the delivery of the health legacy accruing from the Olympic Games in 2012, has published many progress reports on the internet, such as:

- New health strategy to get Londoners more active by 2012
- Experts analyse likely impact of London 2012 on physical activity

There is also an online in-depth analysis written by Barbara Panet-Raymond and David Cooper, entitled *Public Health Legacy: Experiences from Vancouver 2010 and Sydney Olympic and Paralympic Games*. The authors look at legacies which are tangible (such as the use of Olympic venues by the public as facilities for exercise and sport) and intangible, such as the potential to improve collaborative working between a range of government and private organisations.

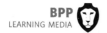

Chapter 4

The justification of this selected topic
History, informed by the events at Hillsborough in 1989 and Munich in 1972, tells us that we cannot be certain that the Games in 2012 will pass smoothly.

Global interest will be intense, not only in the competitions themselves but also in any accompanying incident or outbreak. With regard to the reputation of the health service, the stakes could hardly be higher.

And there is also the possibility of achieving a remarkable public health legacy. In 2009, Dr Simon Tanner, Regional Director of Public Health for London, stated: *'The Games could be the much needed catalyst for a health legacy for all of us – the first the world has seen – but only if we work together to make it happen.'*

Why you find this topic so interesting?
It may be that your enthusiasm for sport led to an ever increasing interest in the risks to health, and the opportunities to promote wellbeing which accompanied the hosting of a huge event like the Olympic Games. In addition, it may have been that, as a result of your reading around the subject, you gained a new understanding of what is meant by 'health' and what might be done to promote good health for communities of people.

Preparation topic 7: What do you think is the most exciting development on the medical horizon?

You really have to be prepared for a question like this. And for you to respond to this question in a manner which suggests that you have never given the matter a second thought will be effectively to give the lie to all your comments about your passion for studying Medicine.

As for the choice of topic, it has to be YOURS and YOURS alone. By asking this question, the interviewer is seeking above all to check just how real your enthusiasm is!

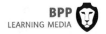

You may have a real interest in technological developments, such as those which now play key parts in surgical operations, or which appear to offer a platform for the construction of artificial organs. Alternatively, you may be absolutely fascinated by medical genetics, and the future possible therapeutic approaches which an increased understanding of the subject may lead to.

For illustrative purposes, let us take as our most exciting development on the medical horizon that of **stem cell research**.

As before, we will look to prepare for the three key lines of inquiry:

Assembling a factual understanding

You have to be ready to demonstrate your knowledge of the subject itself. Indeed, you must welcome the chance.

The interviewer might open the discussions by asking '*So what exactly are stem cells?*'

Now, you don't need to be an expert in the field to be excited by it. You will not be expected to know everything there is to know – but you will be expected to be able to demonstrate your grasp of the basics. And remember, it is a conversation you are preparing for, not an examination. You cannot possibly master every detail relating to 'human-animal hybrid embryos' or 'admixed embryos'. Everyone has limitations to their knowledge, and the important thing is to feel very comfortable in admitting it! You will best demonstrate your understanding of the subject, and at the same time provide evidence of your scholarly approach, by accessing the **scientific literature** for the important facts and definitions. (There are excellent online informative articles from the United States National Institutes of Health at http://stemcells.nih.gov, and at www.newscientist.com/topic/stem-cells.)

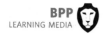

You will find that 'stem cells' are described as cells which have the potential to transform themselves into practically all other types of cells or to revert to being stem cells of even greater reproductive capacity. You will need to be able to describe the distinction between 'adult' stem cells – stem cells which are found in all tissue of the growing human being – and 'embryonic' stem cells found in human embryos, but which are presently obtained at the expense of the life of the embryo.

The interviewer might then explore your understanding of their practical significance. So, prepare by looking first at stem cells' track record of success. For many years, adult stem cells have been used for cancer patients receiving high dose radiotherapy, or chemotherapy, treatments which would normally obliterate the patient's ability to renew their own blood cells. By removing in advance some of their own bone marrow stem cells and then reinjecting them after their cancer treatment, these patients can then resume formation of their blood cells. There have also been case reports that bone marrow stem cells which were injected into an area of damaged heart muscle after a patient suffered a heart attack converted into heart muscle, with consequent improvement in heart function within a few weeks. At the time of writing, the first embryonic stem cell trial in humans to gain approval from regulators in any European country is about to begin at Moorfields Eye Hospital in London. This study will investigate the safety of using retinal pigment cells derived from stem cells to treat people suffering from a rare, incurable, form of macular dystrophy. The researchers believe that while it is just possible for this therapy to reverse the condition, a more realistic hope is that the approach will protect against further loss of sight.

With regard to their possible impacts in the longer term future, hardly a week goes by without a report of some animal or laboratory experiment which indicates a potential future role for stem cells in helping people suffering from a range of medical conditions including certain forms of blindness, multiple sclerosis, diabetes, Alzheimer's disease, Parkinson's disease, and strokes.

Indeed, some researchers believe, based on experiments in rats, that an individual's stem cells may be able to manufacture any of their organs with a blood supply. This ultimately may reduce future need for organ transplantations.

The justification for your selection of this topic

The interviewer has asked you to select a medical topic which you find 'exciting'. There are no objective criteria to which you can turn to convince the panel as to the reasons why YOU are so interested in this subject. If you 'book learn' a reply to this question, you can be sure that the panel will detect that, and they will take a dim view!

Why you find this topic so interesting?

When you explain to someone that you are excited by something, you are telling them about **your personality, and your values**. So, reflect carefully upon these, and be prepared to explain the reality of your position with passion.

Your own viewpoint relating to ethical issues

By reading around the subject, you will appreciate that there are ethical concerns relating to embryonic stem cell research. You can place the issues within the medical ethics framework:

- **Autonomy**
  There are those who believe that human embryonic trials are an assault on the sanctity of the life of the unborn child.

- **Beneficience**
  Some argue that the medical profession's moral duty to cure illness is sufficient justification. Adult stem cell treatments have a proven value; therefore, supporters would say, it is entirely appropriate to engage in a substantial research effort to evaluate the potential effectiveness of embryonic stem cells.

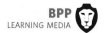

In keeping with this principle, in October 2008 the UK Parliament voted for a series of measures which includes allowing the production of human-animal 'hybrid embryos' for stem cells production, and the creation of 'saviour siblings' to provide bone marrow or umbilical cord tissue for treating genetic conditions.

- **Non-maleficence**
  The destruction of any live embryo flies in the face of this duty to do no harm. And it is noteworthy that, as yet, there is no certainty that such destruction will yield actual practical therapeutic success.

- **Justice**
  Some assert that the social, economic and personal costs of diseases that embryonic stem cells have the potential to treat are far greater than the costs associated with the destruction of embryos.

  There are also those who are concerned about the impact of the legislation which now permits the creation of human-animal 'hybrid embryos' for the purposes of stem cell production. Because of the shortage of human egg cells, human cells are injected into an egg taken from an animal, usually a rabbit. Some fear that this will lead to the development of half-human-half-animal creatures, so called 'humanzees'.

In your preparation, you would need to take the time to reflect upon exactly where you stand. You could well be asked: *'So, do you support embryonic stem cell research, or not?'*. And you would then be invited to explain your position!

The reason behind your own special interest in the subject

It is you who defines what is, or is not, exciting to you!

Certainly, it is perfectly understandable for someone to become very fascinated about this research field because of the huge

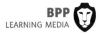

range of medical conditions which might become amenable to treatment by stem cells: this clinical approach truly has the potential to improve the quality of life for millions of people.

And it may also be the case that you have been brought into contact with the effects of stem cell treatment in your own personal or family life.

If you are a rugby player, or indeed a fan of the game, the subject may have been brought to life for you on reading that the South African Rugby World Cup winner Joost van der Westhuizen had, in 2011, begun to undergo experimental stem cell therapy in a bid to slow the progress of the motor neurone disease from which he was suffering.

In summary: for an exciting medical development, try and choose a topic:

- **That really fascinates you**
- **Through which you can enthusiastically demonstrate your factual understanding, and your careful appreciation of related ethical issues**
- **Which also has a personal connection in some way.**

Preparation topic 8: Discussions about management, leadership and teamwork

All doctors are responsible for the use of resources, such as prescription medicines (for example, antibiotics, steroids), operating theatre facilities, and perhaps above all, their own professional time. Many doctors also lead teams, or are involved in teams led by others. To ensure that the expectations and needs of the public are met, all doctors must be actively engaged in the management and leadership of health services. They must also be energetic members of effective teams.

We will now look at these themes: management, leadership, and teamwork, in that order.

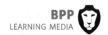

Chapter 4

Imagined question 1

'What is management?'

The General Medical Council's booklet, *Management for Doctors*, is required reading on this subject. The GMC states:

> '. . . management is defined as getting things done well through and with people, creating an environment in which people can perform as individuals and yet co-operate towards achieving group goals, and removing obstacles to such performance.'

In that booklet, it is also stated:

> 'Seven principles have been widely accepted as offering a useful set of principles for doctors who manage. The seven principles are: selflessness; integrity; objectivity; accountability; honesty; openness; leadership.'

In your preparation, reflect upon how each of these seven principles applies to you. And when so doing, write down examples drawn from your own experiences which substantiate these reflections.

Imagined question 2

'What is leadership?'

According to The New Shorter Oxford English Dictionary, one definition of the verb 'to lead' is 'to guide by persuasion as contrasted with commands or threats.' In this regard, 'leadership' is the act of so guiding in practice.

Imagined question 3

'What are the key qualities of a good leader?'

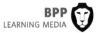

There is much written upon this subject. There is wide consensus that effective leaders:

- Have excellent communication skills; can 'hold court'.
- Radiate confidence and buoyant mood.
- Are visionary in outlook, and also have the courage to reappraise situations and decisions (sometimes their own!) with a fresh critical eye and adapt flexibly and quickly to change.
- Display honesty, integrity, consistency.
- Focus upon actions, outcomes, and completion, not just words.
- Are willing to take responsibility, and possess a mental toughness.
- Are able to motivate, be respected by 'followers' and select good teams.
  But it is not about seeking to be liked. Some highly talented people make ineffective leaders because of their overwhelming need to be liked by everyone.
- Welcome challenges and respect criticisms, and are undaunted by them.
- Are thrilled by the prospect of challenge.

Harvard University has done a lot of research into the key characteristics of the most effective leaders. They have two common qualities. One, which is blindingly obvious, is drive. The other is what they label humility, by which they mean the ability to listen, to admit your own mistakes and to give credit to other people rather than take it all yourself.

Modern healthcare is complex. Doctors have a legal authority broader than any other health professionals; they also have a responsibility to contribute to the running of the organisation within which they work. And, in medical practice, there will also be occasions when it is important for someone used to providing effective leadership to play an excellent support role as a follower.

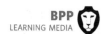

Chapter 4

What does all of this have to do with your medical school interview?

Well, it all goes back to the important criterion for selection: selection for medical school implies selection for the medical profession.

Management and leadership skills are increasingly important qualities for the doctors of the future. So, the panel are looking to see evidence of the following qualities amongst those applying to study Medicine:

- Self awareness; welcoming feedback, knowing when to seek help from others.
- Self-management; respecting the importance of agreed deadlines.
- Self-development.
- Acting with integrity.
- Having the ability to develop networks and relationships.
- Encouraging others within a team.
- Working as a leader and a follower within teams; respecting the skills of others, communicating with clarity and supporting other team members.

Reflect: have there been times when you were a leader? Perhaps you led an expedition, or a hill climbing group. If so, what was the experience like?

What went well; and in what way, exactly did YOU help to make things go well?

What went wrong; and how did YOU help to put things right?

And have there been occasions when you were led by someone else? What did you learn from that?

Important website: www.institute.nhs.uk/medicalleadership

This will give you information about the Enhancing Engagement in Medical Leadership project, a project led by the Academy of Medical Royal Colleges and the NHS Institute. The goal of the project is to create a culture of greater medical engagement in management and leadership among all doctors.

Teamwork

The New Shorter Oxford English Dictionary defines 'team' as 'a group of people collaborating in their professional work' and 'teamwork' as 'combined action of a group of people, especially when effective and efficient'.

In healthcare, good, effective teamwork is essential to success. For example, there is an amazing sense of 'pulling together' when surgeons, anaesthetists, and nurses collectively manage a complex case in operating theatre.

But teamwork does not always come easily. Some commentators divide people into those who are either 'givers' or 'takers': it seems as if there are always going to be occasions when the 'idle' rely on the energy and enthusiasm of the committed.

So, one of the key challenges to any team is make sure that *everyone* pulls their weight.

Teams work best when all members share a clear understanding of the overall goals. A good team member:

- Respects and supports the contributions of ALL colleagues.
  - Lack of respect for colleagues, for example, by patronising them, ignoring them, or disrespecting them, may affect the quality of care.
- Communicates effectively within and outside the team.
- Ensures that others understand their role and responsibilities, and they also understand the roles and responsibilities of

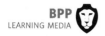

others. (There is clarity around 'who does what?' and 'who leads on what?')

- Accepts their responsibilities, and is reliable.

A good team leader also makes sure that:

- All team members are clear about the team objectives and their own role in meeting those objectives.
- All members of the team are given timely opportunities to discuss situations.
- Lessons are learnt from experiences, especially from mistakes.

For example, the following have been shown to be 'markers' of effective team meetings:

- Members do not talk over each other.
- Everybody is encouraged to contribute to the meeting.
- A sense of humour is encouraged.
- Key pertinent questions are raised, and related issues considered.

One important example of the team approach in Medicine is the development of multidisciplinary teams (MDTs) caring for patients with cancer.

Multidisciplinary clinical teams are made up of professionals from those specialties which are involved in providing care for patients suffering from specific conditions. For example, an MDT for patients with bowel cancer will obtain membership from surgeons, anaesthetists, dieticians, physiotherapists, nurses, psychiatrists and oncologists. The aim of the team, usually (but not always) led by a consultant surgeon, is to establish the best treatment plan for the individual patient. The successful MDT will ensure that the patient, and their family, have confidence that all their clinical needs are attended to, that care is co-ordinated, and that options which appear to offer an improved outcome are fully and carefully considered.

Another example of effective teamwork in practice is the 'Hospital at Night' initiative. (See Glossary.)

Possible questions on teamwork:

- *'What makes a good team member?'*
- *'Can you give an example of how you played a successful part in a team?'*
- *'Have you ever been part of a team when the objectives were not met? Why was this? What did you learn from the experience?'*

Preparation topic 9: Discussions about the importance of teaching

The word 'doctor' is derived from the Latin word 'docere' meaning *to teach*. It is a requirement that all medical students develop and demonstrate basic teaching skills and are willing to contribute to the education of other students.

During their course, medical students will be expected to develop the skills, attitudes and practices of a competent teacher.

In recent years, interview panels have increasingly sought to obtain a picture of the applicant's approach to teaching. Do you relish the opportunity; or is it an ordeal?

So, as part of your preparation, reflect carefully upon your own experience in this field. For example, at home, have you helped to teach your younger brothers and sisters in Mathematics? At school, have you ever been asked to help correct younger pupils' science homework? How did you find these experiences? What did you learn about yourself as a teacher?

Let us imagine this possible question from the panel.

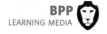

Chapter 4

Imagined question

> *'You have been asked to lead a one-hour session in which a group of six 14-year-old children are to be taught the basics of atomic structure. How would you do this?'*

You may have done something like this before, in which case you are well placed to reflect upon the experience: what went well, and what did not go so well?

There are also some very helpful on line articles and reports which can help you to frame your response: for example, the General Medical Council's document *The Doctor as Teacher*, and the paper from the BMA entitled *Doctors as Teachers*.

You can think about planning for this session by breaking it down into three key components.

- **Scope the subject matter** to be covered, and **agree the session's aims**
- Decide which **educational approach** you will adopt when conducting the session, and
- **Evaluate the impact of the session, by both giving and receiving feedback.**

Let us look at each of these in turn.

Scoping what is to be covered; agreeing the session's aims

The topic to be taught is defined in the imagined question: the basics of atomic structure. The next step would be for you to set the **key aims** of the session. This is best done in consultation with members of the class. You could start by finding out in broad terms how much each of them already knows about the subject. For example, are they familiar with the concept that all matter comprises of chemical elements? Having heard from the group, you would then be in a position to explain what you intend to cover in the session:

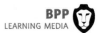

'By the end of the session, the group will have gained an understanding of the concept of how all matter is made up of around one hundred different kinds of substances, elements, each of which cannot be broken down by chemical means into anything simpler; and that any quantity of an element is made up of tiny "building bricks", called atoms; and that elements are distinguished from each other fundamentally by the structure of their atoms, the atom of each element having its own unique nuclear and electronic configuration.'

Conducting the session: the educational approach

You will need to decide upon the teaching style you wish to adopt. Would you favour a didactic approach, in which the children would almost entirely spend the time listening to you? Or would you be keen to obtain their involvement – after all, there is only going to be six of them: in this way you would be acting more as a leader of discussions than a formal teacher.

Evaluating the impact of the session; obtaining and receiving feedback

Whichever approach you were to take, it will be important to gauge the level of success you have achieved by the end of the session. And there are two aspects to this feedback. Firstly, it will be important to measure the level of success you will have had in communicating an understanding of these basics to each child. However, secondly, perhaps more importantly, in order that *you* also can learn from the session, there is the need to know how it felt for them; how much did they enjoy the session, and what aspects were they not so keen on?

Preparation time spent in gaining some insight into teaching methods, and into how we all learn in our different ways, is time very well spent. Why not ask one of your science teachers to tell you how they prepare for a new term's syllabus?

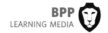

You don't have to become an expert in the field. However, it is crucial that you are able to engage with the panel around your own approach to teaching, a subject which is of increasing significance when it comes to selecting medical students.

KEY POINTS

- Facts are important, but your interview goes far beyond an assessment of your factual understanding.
- Reflect upon your judgements, and the criteria which justify them.
- Believe in yourself, and in the values you hold dear: they have served you well so far.
- Make your preparation for the interview *fun* – enjoy it!
- You cannot possibly become an expert on every topic or theme: so *focus* on a few areas, and read around the subjects.
- Practise, practise, practise, but don't over rehearse!
- Prepare to be natural!

Chapter 5

Mature and graduate students

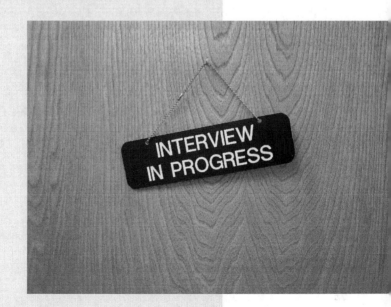

Mature and graduate students

Our working definition of a mature student is someone over the age of 21 applying to study at university for the first time.

For any mature student, there is apprehension about the length of time which has elapsed since they were last in full-time education. There may well also be concerns around the financial implications of giving up work.

But, while it cannot be said that starting medical studies when you are older is easy, that should not put anyone off if they have absolutely made their mind up that a medical career is the one for them.

Certainly, it is the case that many mature students begin, and complete, their medical studies every year.

For graduate applicants who have completed a first degree in another subject, it will be important for them to reflect very carefully upon why they have now decided to study Medicine. Completing the medical degree means spending at least seven years as a student; seven years of not being out there in the workplace!

Having received their letters inviting them to interview, it is vital that mature and graduate applicants enter into the process feeling wholly unapologetic about their situation. Yes, they now want to study Medicine with a real passion: but that simply does not mean that their earlier decisions were in any way 'errors of judgement'. One of the key principles of 'lifelong learning' is that we must acknowledge all the positive aspects of whatever we do in life.

At interview, the panel will apply all the university's assessment criteria for selection to medical school which we looked at in Chapter 3 of this book.

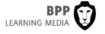

However, as a mature or graduate applicant, you must particularly prepare to discuss the following themes with the panel:

- Your motivation for, and commitment to, studying Medicine NOW. What has happened to you to lead you into this choice? Will you complete the course?
- Your experience of the real world. Has it helped you to strengthen your interpersonal skills? If so, how? Has it helped you to take responsibility? In what specific areas?

Many mature and graduate students who have gone on to complete their medical studies have been much more self-directed, challenging, and questioning than their younger colleagues. They have already learnt how to study, to take responsibility for their own educational development.

- What can you bring to the medical course? Again, experience has shown that mature and graduate students often enter Medicine with a high level of related knowledge which can be very valuable to other students, especially within the problem-based learning setting. Many are able to broaden the richness of the educational experience of the course, especially those coming from a background outside science.
- How will you feel when studying alongside younger students, and then working, and competing for positions, with them? Will you be comfortable?
- How will you handle the temptations attached to student life, and adjust to the challenges of changes to your financial and domestic situations?

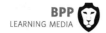

KEY POINTS

- Before submitting your application, contact the medical schools and find out about their requirements and opportunities.
- Speak to someone who is already studying Medicine as a mature or graduate student.
- What advice do they give?

And prepare for the questions:

- Why did you not study Medicine the first time around?
- Knowing what you know now, what would you do if you had your time again?
- You are moving on from your first choice: will you move on from Medicine? Is it all a pipe-dream too far?

Chapter 6

Your performance on the day

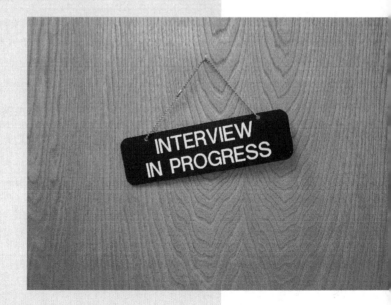

Your performance on the day

Just like your driving test, or first A level examination, the day of your medical school interview will bring feelings of nervous agitation and the hope that it will soon, all be over so that life can go back to normal!

But don't lose sight of the big picture: your interview provides the one key opportunity for you to be at the very centre of events regarding your application to study Medicine.

Yes, it will be stressful. Interviews are stressful *for everyone!*

So, try to relax in ways which you know work for you and take heart from knowing that you have prepared thoroughly. But don't strain to become someone you are simply not. It is vital that your real, unique personality comes through on the day!

Prepare for your journey carefully, and aim to arrive early (but not too early) and certainly not too late. Imagine how you would handle some 'worst scenarios'. What would you do if, for example, having set off, you simply couldn't get there on time? Whatever else, make sure that you can contact the medical school to let them know what has happened. They will almost certainly offer you another date.

Psychologically, it might be helpful for you to take a couple of examples of evidence of any special achievements, or of material you have assembled as part of your preparation which has special significance for you.

Key fact: The interview begins as soon as you come into the view of members of the medical school staff; it ends when you have left and you are out of sight. If you are greeted by a medical student, just remember they may well be invited to give feedback to the panel.

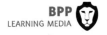

So be courteous, pleasant and polite to everyone you meet!

Your appearance

Like it or not, it is a fact that the members of the panel will look at how you are dressed and groomed. Are you someone they would be pleased to have looking after their families?

The conventional advice is: 'dress for success'. This entails looking smart and comfortable. Keep your choice of jewellery, make up and hair style simple. Your shoes need not be new, but they do need to be clean and polished.

And check your finger nails!

Your verbal performance; what you say and what you do not say

Try to vary your conversational style in both its grammatical structure and the modulation of your voice; to be one dimensional is to appear dull and uninteresting.

Don't go on and on: try to build up your replies carefully. The most effective responses are usually four or five sentences in length, making no more than three points in reply to each question. So, try not to explain everything you know about a topic in one long speech!

Be precise in your language; don't use jargon, clichés, acronyms and abbreviations. And be assertive, not apologetic or defensive: it is important that you do not let the interviewer obtain the wrong impression of what you say. You must defend your point of view, but always in a reasonable tone. Coming over as sincere, honest and trustworthy goes a long way.

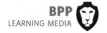

Establishing rapport

The skill is to relate to all members of the panel when answering every question. People who are interested in each other make eye contact when they speak to confirm that they really are being listened to. So, if you don't look at someone when you are speaking to them, don't be surprised if they appear to 'switch off' and seem not to be interested in what you have to say. They may well have come to feel that by not looking at them you are signalling that you are not interested in them, nor in their reaction to your comments. And when any of us feel uninvolved, our concentration lapses.

Your non-verbal performance

The manner in which you present yourself, and how you speak, is also of vital importance.

Some research has indicated that the results of many interviews are decided within the first few minutes of the candidate's arrival in the room, and these decisions are often made instinctively. If true, this adds even greater significance to the non-verbal aspects of your performance at interview, such as your mood, attitude and demeanour. Your body language, especially your facial expression, tells the panel a great deal about how you feel inside at any point in time. So, smile when you enter the interview room, and make sure your opening handshakes are firm, indicating that you are pleased to be there.

You must demonstrate respect for the members of the panel, and at the same time be confident in your manner. Certainly, this is not the occasion for any displays of arrogance. Try not to be put off by members of the panel taking notes during your discussions. You simply have to accept that they will be sharing their views upon your performance afterwards, and they need to be able to evidence their own opinions and perspectives.

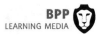

Don't fiddle with your watch, or any other jewellery. Above all, try to enjoy every minute of it rather than give the appearance that you are enduring one of the biggest ordeals of your life!

Your final impression

You will almost certainly be offered the following opportunity by the panel.

Imagined question

'So far, we have asked you the questions. Is there anything **YOU** *would like to ask the panel?'*

As we have seen before, the skill is to make the words mean what you want to them mean. So in response to this invitation you have to be prepared to SAY something.

This is your chance to leave a final impression that makes a mark, and to ensure that you do not leave the interview room with any sense of regret.

Of course it is not the time for you to ask something just for the sake of it – the panel will take a dim view of that. So, if you really feel that everything has been covered fully, then take the opportunity to say so as politely and sincerely as possible; and make sure that you sound as though you have enjoyed the experience!

Alternatively, you could:

- Seek to clarify aspects of the course which very much attract you, such as the possibility of conducting research, or of spending some time abroad, or of obtaining an intercalated degree. Here is your chance to find out if the course on offer is the one best suited to yourself.
- Take this opportunity not to ask any questions, but to clarify something you said during the interview; you might have

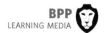

suddenly remembered a salient fact, for example. To do this demonstrates your pride in your performance, and that would not be lost on the panel.

(But make just one point; you cannot revise your entire performance!)

What do interviewers talk about after you have gone?

When you have finally taken your leave of the interview panel and walk away from the university buildings, your head will be spinning with it all: there will be parts of the interview that went really well, but you will also be wishing you had said some things instead of others.

As for the interviewers, well given that no two sets of panel members are the same you can be sure that their discussions will vary too. However, we do know they will discuss your performance with regard to the assessment criteria, and then inform the admissions tutors of their overall judgement.

It is our experience that when describing the performance of candidates who have interviewed successfully, panel members are far more likely to use words such as 'natural', 'enthusiastic', 'fluent', and 'bright' about them.

This is entirely in keeping with their focus being so much more upon your *personality* and your *ability to engage* than your memory and factual recall.

For the panel to describe such candidates as 'knowledgable' is rare indeed!

Equally, when commenting upon candidates who are not recommended for selection, words such as 'boring', 'uninteresting', 'uninspiring' and, notably, 'rehearsed' are those which are often used.

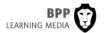

KEY POINTS

Your mission on the day is to convince the panel that, having thought about your future very carefully:

- You are passionately keen, and determined, to study Medicine.
- You are very keen to study at that medical school.
- You know what is required of you if you are accepted, and
- You have what it takes to succeed; in completing the course and then becoming a good doctor.

So, make sure that you:

- Concentrate
- Listen carefully, and
- Stay enthusiastic and spirited *whatever happens*.

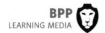

Chapter 7

Final thoughts

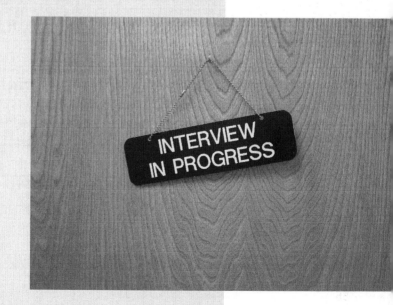

Final thoughts

To restate the obvious: there is no such thing as a standard medical school interview. Despite all your efforts, you may still be taken by surprise at some of the panel's questions.

However, have no doubt; the time you spend upon preparation is time well spent. And this doesn't mean absorbing fact after fact after fact! It is much more about getting ready to justify *everything* you say. So, make sure you have your examples, think about the criteria which support your judgements, and feel comfortable about yourself and your values.

In particular, take confidence from the way you have prepared for discussions on the current and future challenges to the health service, and on medical developments. By staying abreast of issues as they develop, and then reading the relevant, authoritative scientific and political reports, you demonstrate the qualities of diligence, scholarship, enthusiasm and curiosity, qualities which the interviewers are so keen to explore in candidates for medical schools.

In closing, we would list some 'things to avoid' and a few 'top tips'.

Medical school interview: things to avoid

- Not having visited the university before.
- Arriving for the interview late; rushing.
- Forgetting the content of your personal statement.
- Appearing over-rehearsed.
- Trying to be funny; being glib, casual or uninterested.
- Dishonesty; deliberately misleading the panel.
- Using any word or phrase the meaning of which you are uncertain.

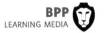

- Using acronyms, especially those with which panel members are likely to be unfamiliar, and very especially if you don't know the meaning yourself!
- Drying up completely, BUT there are times when silence is very powerful.
- Using tentative language, such as:
'I think I might do . . .';
But it is perfectly acceptable to start a response by saying, 'I am not certain what I would do because every situation / patient is unique. However, I know the things that I would be considering are . . .'
- Fudging. If you don't know the answer to a factual question, then admit it and get ready to move on.
- Drawing attention to any weakness UNLESS you are learning from it, handling it, and becoming a more complete person.
- Criticising others; casting yourself in a favourable light compared to others.
- Interrupting the panel; arguing with the panel.
But be prepared to disagree politely and sincerely.
- Answering the wrong question; answering a question you would like to be asked rather than one you are asked.
- Asking the interviewer to re-phrase a question. Why should they?
But by all means seek clarity if you are genuinely unsure
- Being passive, apologetic; being aggressive
- Lacking enthusiasm, sincerity and vitality.

Medical school interview: top tips

- Ensure you have a good night's sleep the night before.
- Consider your appearance; dress, hair, shoes, finger nails.
- Arrive early, but not too early.
- Rehearse your entrance, especially your first handshake.
- Smile
- Be mindful of your body language.
- Concentrate; don't let your nerves stop you hearing what is being said.

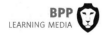

- Listen carefully; and show the panel that you are listening.
- Practise being assertive.
- Vary the tone of your voice.
- See yourself as preparing to RESPOND to the panel's questions rather than formulating answers to them.
- Engage with all panel members.
- Keep your responses to four or five sentences, then wait and listen.
- PREPARE and PRACTISE with your family, friends, teachers.
- Smile.
  Be honest about yourself, but also be kind to yourself!

Post script: after the interview

This will not be the only interview you will have in your life.

Indeed, you may well have other interviews before you find out whether or not you have been offered a place at medical school.

It is vital that we learn from all our experiences. So, beginning the following day, write down your memories of the day; try to record the subjects which were covered.

And reflect particularly upon:

- How could you prepare better?
- What could you have done differently on the day?

Then, design an action plan to improve your performance at your next interview!

We strongly recommend that you do seek more information from medical school websites and advice from staff at the medical school you wish to attend to ensure that you become as well prepared as possible for your medical school interview.

Chapter 8

Glossary of further medical terms

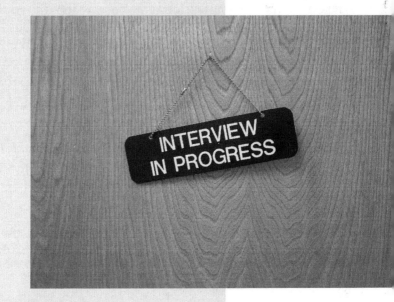

Glossary of further medical terms

British Medical Association

The British Medical Association (BMA) is the voluntary independent trade union and professional association for medical students and doctors of all branches of medicine in the United Kingdom. The BMA seeks to maintain the honour and interests of the medical profession and promote the achievement of high quality healthcare.

The BMA formulates policies on public health issues, medical ethics, the state of the National Health Service and medical education; BMA members have access to one of the finest medical libraries in the UK.

The BMA Careers Service provides members with tools and skills to manage and develop a successful career in the medical profession.

Care Quality Commission

The Care Quality Commission is the body within the government of the United Kingdom, established in 2009, which regulates and inspects health and social care services, including the National Health Service, in England. The Commission is responsible for assuring safety and quality, and for assessing the performance of healthcare commissioners (Primary Care Trusts) and providers (NHS hospital Trusts).

The Commission also has powers of enforcement towards ensuring compliance with regulatory requirements.

Clinical audit

Clinical audit embraces the systematic critical analysis of the quality of clinical care whereby the actual professional performance (including the analysis of the procedures used for diagnosis and treatment, the use of healthcare resources, and the resulting outcome and quality of life of the patient) of a **clinical team, or department,** is compared to an agreed standard for such performance.

Clinical audit seeks to identify deficiencies in a team's performance so that they may be remedied. The aim is for the team to improve its standard of care for patients.

Example: The National Service Framework (NSF) for Coronary Heart Disease sets out a standard for the time taken for patients suffering a heart attack to receive clot dissolving treatment (thrombolysis); namely, that all patients eligible for thrombolysis should receive that treatment within one hour of calling for professional help.

An example of a clinical audit study in a hospital cardiology department would be to:

- Identify the proportion of people receiving such treatment who were actually treated within one hour of calling for professional help, and

- Set out, and implement, recommendations designed to raise this proportion to the required standard of 100 per cent.

  In 2007/8, nationally, about 71 per cent of people treated with thrombolysis received their treatment within 60 minutes.

Clinical governance

Clinical governance is the term used to describe a systematic approach to maintaining and improving the quality of patient care within a health **system, such as a hospital**. The most widely used formal definition is:

> *'A framework through which NHS organisations are accountable for continually improving the quality of their services and*

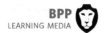

> *safeguarding high standards of care by creating an environment in which excellence in clinical care will flourish.' (Scally and Donaldson, 1998)*

In essence, clinical governance means that everyone working within the NHS should feel a strong sense of personal responsibility towards the maintenance of the highest standards of healthcare and ensuring that mistakes are dealt with and lessons learnt.

Clinical research

The key goal for any clinical research is to identify a new way of treating, or preventing, a disease or condition. This new information can then be made available for the benefit of all who suffer, or who may in future suffer, from that disease or condition.

Clinical research may be carried out by epidemiological and intervention studies.

Epidemiological studies

Epidemiology is the study of the distribution and determinants of disease frequency in man.

An interesting example is the Framingham Study. The health experiences of just over 5,000 men and women who lived in the town of Framingham, Massachusetts, were studied for several decades from shortly after the end of the Second World War. This study showed that people who smoked regularly, had high levels of blood cholesterol and raised blood pressure were at increased risk of heart disease.

Intervention studies

Intervention studies look at how changes in situations affect health.

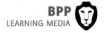

For example, consider the study of the impact of treating raised blood pressure on the future likelihood of suffering from a stroke. The UK Medical Research Council conducted such as study in the 1980s: some people with raised blood pressure received treatment over a period of time, while others of the same age did not receive such treatment. The numbers of strokes occurring in the two groups of people were then compared; the number of people suffering strokes in the treated group were considerably fewer than in those not treated.

Analysing the effectiveness of a new surgical approach, such as transplantation, is another important kind of intervention study.

Clinical trials are a special form of intervention study. This kind of research looks to see if a new drug, or vaccine, has an impact upon the number of cases of a condition, or in some way reduces the severity of the condition.

Before any research study is carried out, there needs to be consideration of:

- Risks: foreseeable risks must not outweigh expected benefits.
- Ethical issues. This is especially the case if the study aims to assess the effectiveness of a clinical approach in managing a condition by comparing outcomes in a 'treated' group of patients suffering from the condition with outcomes in a 'non-treated' group of such patients. It would be ethically unacceptable to deny patients a therapy which is believed to be effective simply in order to conduct a research project.

Not all doctors in the NHS carry out research projects.

However, results from research studies are the basis of 'Evidence-based medicine' (see below).

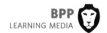

Accordingly, all doctors should obtain a clear understanding of the principles of research so as to be able to take a view upon the significance of the results presented.

Continuing Professional Development

All doctors are responsible for identifying their educational requirements and then ensuring that they are met.

Continuing Professional Development (CPD) is a professional obligation on doctors who have completed their postgraduate education.

CPD requires them to:

- Further develop and maintain the knowledge, skills and attributes which are necessary for good medical practice, and
- Embrace proven improvements in their field.

The Royal Colleges set standards for yearly CPD achievements and they award appropriate educational courses study-time based credits.

CPD will form an important component of the system whereby the licence to practice for all doctors will be revalidated.

Lifelong learning

Lifelong learning is an educational philosophy which increasingly underpins CPD by encouraging all doctors to be open to new ideas and the acquisition of new skills. The ethos of lifelong learning promotes partnerships between different professional groups, such as between doctors and nurses, with the aim of facilitating learning experiences across and within the multi-professional clinical fields.

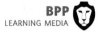

In its document, *Tomorrow's Doctors* the General Medical Council recommends that medical schools' curricula should 'foster the knowledge and understanding, attitudes and skills that will promote lifelong learning and support professional development'.

Department of Health

The Department of Health (DoH) is a department of the government of the United Kingdom. It is led by the Secretary for State for Health, supported by a junior ministerial team.

The DoH is responsible for government health policy and is directly responsible for the NHS in England through Strategic Health Authorities. (Scotland, Wales and Northern Ireland have their own local administrations).

Epidemic

An epidemic is a widespread occurrence of a disease in a community at a particular time.

European Working Time Directive

The European Working Time Directive is a collection of regulations concerning hours of work; the Directive is designed to protect the health and safety of the work force. The Directive was enshrined in UK law in 1998 and on 1st August, 2009, it was fully applied to junior doctors – reducing the maximum number of hours worked from, on average, 56 per week to 48. The implementation of the Directive has been instrumental in the NHS adopting new ways of working, including:

* Directing medical staff into day time working.
* Developing split site services: such as having Out-patient and Day Case services for a local population being carried out in one hospital, and Emergency and Inpatients for the same population cared for in a different hospital.

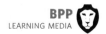

- Developing the role of specialist nurses and nurse practitioners, who are able to assume responsibility for some duties formerly carried out by doctors.
- Developing new posts, such as clinical technicians and clinical assistant practitioner posts.

Euthanasia

How sacred is life? How can anyone know whether life has become intolerable for someone?

High profile cases, where the outcome is governed by a High Court judge, serve to remind us all of the complexity of decision-making for patients who suffer from serious life threatening disease.

Some people believe that life, seemingly any sort of life, is always better than death. Within the medical profession, there are those who place great emphasis upon treating clinical conditions, sometimes to the exclusion of recognising that, for the suffering patient, death might be a more welcome outcome.

Others recognise that there are circumstances in which the continuation of medical attempts to prolong life are either clearly futile or inflict unbearable suffering, and that there are occasions when there is a strong case for enabling a patient to refuse treatment which prolongs a life wholly lacking in quality.

Definitions

Euthanasia: the deliberate killing of a person for the benefit of that person, to reduce pain or suffering.

Mercy killing: the act of killing someone who suffers from an incurable disease in a painless way.

In the United Kingdom, the acts of euthanasia and mercy killing constitute murder or manslaughter.

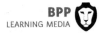

Assisted suicide: a common term for actions by which a person helps someone else take their own life by providing, for example, drugs or equipment. Where doctors are involved in helping a suffering patient to take this action, the term is 'physician assisted suicide'.

In the United Kingdom, the Suicide Act of 1961 makes it illegal to aid, abet, counsel or procure the suicide of another person. The offence carries a maximum prison sentence of 14 years.

However:

- A centre for assisted suicide in Switzerland has helped 100 Britons to die.
- 'Living wills', which are statements made by adults who declare in advance that they would not wish to be kept alive if they became incapacitated or unable to communicate, have legal status in the UK.
- Increasingly, hospital medical and nursing staff engage with individual patients and their carers to consider the patient's status with regard to 'For resuscitation' or 'Do not resuscitate (DNR)'.
- Elderly people and the terminally ill will get the right to choose to die at home instead of in hospital under the terms of Lord Darzi's 2008 NHS review.
- In the light of Debbie Purdy's legal case in 2008, in February 2010, Keir Starmer QC, the Director of Public Prosecutions, announced guidelines which, although not amounting to a change in the law, detailed a set of mitigating factors which weighed against an individual being prosecuted for assisting the suicide of another person. Key amongst these factors is that the suspect was motivated by compassion and that they reported the suicide to the police and fully assisted in their inquiries.

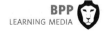

Evidence-based medicine

Evidence-based medicine is clinical practice which is informed by the integration of:

- Best research evidence
- The experience of the doctor's clinical expertise, and
- The patient's values.

Best research must be patient centred, precise and accurate.

The strongest research evidence in support of a clinical intervention comes from well designed controlled trials. In contrast, patients' accounts, individual case reports and expert opinions are considered to provide weaker evidence because of associated biases and subjectivity.

However, there are situations where it would not be appropriate to investigate the impact of a clinical approach by trials which compare the effects of a specific treatment for a condition with the effects of no such treatment. For example, it would be considered to be highly unethical to analyse the impact of antibiotics upon the outcome of patients suffering from pneumonia by means of such a controlled trial. Clinical observation over many years has convinced the medical profession of the importance of such drugs in managing this condition.

Clinical expertise enables the physician to rapidly identify the unique health status of each patient, and the individual risks they face.

Patients' personal values are their own preferences, concerns and expectations.

The integration of these three elements provides the basis of a diagnostic and therapeutic approach which optimises clinical outcomes and quality of life.

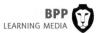

The Cochrane Library

The Cochrane Library contains high-quality, independent evidence to inform healthcare decision-making. It includes reliable evidence from Cochrane and other systematic reviews, clinical trials and more. Cochrane reviews bring together in one report the combined results of the world's best medical research studies, and are recognised as the gold standard in evidence-based healthcare.

General Medical Council

Established in 1858, the General Medical Council is the body which regulates the medical profession in the United Kingdom. It licenses doctors to practise. The key role for the GMC is to protect, promote and maintain high standards of medical practice. The GMC is responsible for deciding the knowledge, skills and attitudes graduates in Medicine need. The principal statement of guidance to doctors issued by the GMC is contained within the document *Good Medical Practice*. This outlines the standards of clinical practice which are expected by the public.

Globesity

The World Health Organisation began commenting upon the rapidly increasing numbers of obese people across the world in the 1990s. And the epidemic is not restricted to industrialised nations; there is evidence of ever increasing numbers of obese people amongst the populations of developing countries. In the UK, it is estimated that the prevalence of obesity has trebled since 1980.

Studies have indicated that obesity predisposes to the development of heart disease, high blood pressure, stroke disease and some forms of cancer, such as cancer of the breast, womb and prostate. There is also evidence that obesity predisposes to kidney failure and the need for dialysis and renal transplantation.

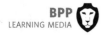

More newborn babies die in Britain than anywhere else in Western Europe, with maternal obesity a significant factor.

The problem now affects children perhaps even more than adults, so that, for example, we now see onset of non-insulin dependent diabetes in children, something which was until recently unknown.

There appears to be two main causal factors: the overeating of foods high in fats and sugars, taken together with an increasing prevalence of inactive lifestyles.

Recent initiatives aimed at impacting on this problem have included:

- A focus on healthier eating in schools.
- A call for the banning of junk food advertisements which target children, and banning the opening of fast food restaurants near schools.
- Promoting the benefits of regular exercise, such as daily walks, and the increased provision of parks and bicycle paths in new housing development plans.
- Offering overweight people cash incentives to lose weight.

There are also reports of the effects of:

- Gastric clamping surgery.
- The potential to develop 'exercise pills', pharmacological agents which stimulate fat reduction.

Health

World Health Organisation definition: 'Health is a state of complete physical, mental and social wellbeing and not merely the absence of disease or infirmity.'

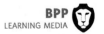

Health Economics

Economic appraisal is concerned with the need to make choices about how scarce resources are used. Resources are scarce in the sense that they will always be insufficient to enable individuals or society to pursue all the objectives they might desire. Accepting this notion means that choice is inevitable.

Economic appraisals are carried out using a systematic framework for identifying and organising the information required for decision-making. All factors impacting on a decision are taken into account, and where possible quantified and valued.

The economic appraisals of alternative healthcare programmes (prevention or treatment) are carried out using three techniques:

* *Cost-benefit analysis*
* *Cost-effectiveness analysis*
* *Cost-utility analysis*

Cost-benefit analysis

This technique compares the costs and outcomes of any programme when both the costs and the outcomes are measured in money.

Cost-effectiveness analysis

Cost-effectiveness analysis refers to the evaluation of a health initiative by measuring the costs incurred and the effects of the initiative in terms of its production of a defined clinical outcome.

For example, the cost-effectiveness of a breast cancer screening programme could be measured calculating the service costs per tumour detected.

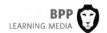

Cost-utility analysis

If it is accepted that the goal of all health service initiatives is to improve the health status of people, there is considerable merit in developing a general measure which would allow changes in health status over time to be quantified.

The cost-utility analysis of a healthcare programme is the methodology by which monetary costs associated with the programme are compared to the programme outcomes, these outcomes being measured in changes in units of health status.

Increasingly, the standard unit of health status used in cost-utility analysis is the 'Quality Adjusted Life Year'.

Quality Adjusted Life Year (QALY)

The outcomes from medical treatments and preventative approaches have two components: the impact upon people's *length of life*, and the impact upon their *quality of life*. The QALY embraces both of these components; it is the arithmetic product of life expectancy and a measure of the quality of the remaining years of life. There are five dimensions of quality within this definition, relating to an individual's:

- Mobility
- Pain and discomfort
- Ability to self-care
- Anxiety and depression
- Ability to carry out usual activities.

So, one QALY equals one year of perfect health, or two years of 50% health, or four years of 25% health.

QALYs are a far from perfect measure of outcome. However, their use when considering resource allocation decisions means that choices between patient groups competing for medical care can be made explicit, and commissioners given an insight into the likely benefits of investing in new technologies and therapies.

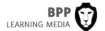

Health promotion

Health promotion includes:

- The provision of information to individuals, families and communities which makes a positive contribution to their health status.
- The motivation of individuals to adopt healthy lifestyles.
- The process of enabling people to increase control over, and to improve, their health.

There are three key strategies underpinning the delivery of health promotion:

- Advocacy for health.
- Enabling all people to achieve their full health potential.
- Mediating between different interests in society towards obtaining an overall improvement in the health of people.

Health Protection Agency

The Health Protection Agency is a non-departmental public body having as its key function the protection of the people of England against infectious diseases and the dangers to health posed by radiation, chemical and environmental hazards. The Agency also provides support to all government departments in co-ordinated and consistent UK public health responses to national level emergencies.

The Agency carries out its responsibilities by providing:

- Advice to local professionals who have health protection duties.
- Training to doctors, nurses and emergency services.
- Co-ordinated exercises at local and national level to improve readiness for major incidents and emergencies.

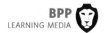

- Surveillance reports, at national and international level, of potential threats.
- Operational lead for 'port health' arrangements.

Hospital at Night (HAN)

The term 'Hospital at Night' entered regular usage when, in 2004, initiatives based on arrangements which were new to the NHS were introduced towards:

- Reducing the long working hours of junior doctors, and
- Meeting requirements of the European Working Time Directive.

'Hospital at Night' is designed around one or more multi-disciplinary teams; each team possesses the full range of skills required to manage all patients' needs during the overnight period.

Features of HAN are:

- Wherever safely possible, giving responsibilities which had been previously carried by medical staff to non-medical professionals within the HAN team, especially nurses.
- Extending the conventional 'working day' to reduce clinical workload at night.
- Reducing unnecessary duplication of effort.
- Assembling teams on the basis of achieving the mix of required competencies rather than focusing upon the grades of staff.
- Providing particularly careful attention to patients' care at times of handover between night staff and wards' day staff.

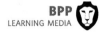

Human Genome Project (HGP)

The HGP was a 13-year long, multinational collaborative initiative, which began in 1990 and was co-ordinated by the US Department of Energy and the US National Institutes of Health. One of the main aims of the project was to gain as full an understanding as possible of the part played by genetic factors in the development of human diseases, so that effective strategies for their diagnosis, treatment and prevention can be devised.

Some diseases, cystic fibrosis for example, are caused by abnormalities affecting one specific gene. However, there are many conditions which can be caused by the abnormalities of several genes and these can be inherited in several ways. There is also a range of conditions – including some forms of heart disease and cancer – which develop as a result of the interaction between a person's genetic constitution and their lifestyle and environment.

In the light of the results of the HGP, scientists are now able to build a clearer picture of the diseases to which any of us are individually prone by identifying whether we possess the genes which are associated with them.

So, as well as being able to test for the likelihood of the future development of specific conditions such as cystic fibrosis, muscular dystrophy and Huntington's disease, a person's susceptibility to other diseases – such as breast cancer – can also be assessed. It is also believed that for couples for whom there are concerns around fertility, the chances of achieving pregnancy will be improved by the ability to select those embryos who have the best chance of developing normally.

However, there are clear ethical issues to consider: for example, with regard to confidentiality on those occasions when sensitive information is revealed about the genetic traits of someone – perhaps a person at higher risk of a chronic but non lethal disease, such as rheumatoid arthritis, say – before they were

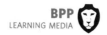

adults and in any position to give consent. And some find something distasteful about pre-selecting children to a pre-determined specification.

Information emerging from the HGP also holds the promise of helping researchers refine drug treatments so that they become more targeted and cause fewer side effects.

Some argue that to discover that they have a higher than average chance of developing a disease serves to motivate an individual to adopt positive lifestyle changes.

However, placed in some hands, this information may lead to the discrimination of some people, possibly groups of people. Some affected individuals may have to pay high life insurance premiums, or even, possibly, fail to obtain life insurance at all.

The UK Genetic Testing Network advises the NHS towards ensuring the provision of high quality genetic testing services for the population of the whole country. This network is supported by laboratory scientists, medical geneticists and representatives from patient support groups.

UK Genetic Testing Network website: www.ukgtn.nhs.uk

Lord Darzi – review of the NHS

The report of Lord Darzi's review of the NHS was published in the week of the 60th anniversary of the NHS, in July 2008.

This report provided a 10-year vision for the further development of the NHS, and focused particularly on the need to increase the quality of individual clinical care and to provide patients with greater choices.

The author stated that: 'The patient experience is the most powerful lever and will be used for service improvement. The

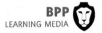

whole report is about quality – it is what energises staff in the NHS.'

Key recommendations from the review which have already been taken forward include:

- To develop a new web-portal whereby the latest clinical and non-clinical evidence of best practice can be assessed.

  'NHS Evidence' was launched in 2009, and is managed by NICE. This is an internet service providing authoritative evidence of best practice.

- Patients with lifelong conditions, such as diabetes, will be able to control their own treatment budgets.

  In December 2011, over 1,300 patients from across the country (particularly those with continuing care needs, and patients suffering from mental health problems) are piloting this initiative.

Medical School Charter

This charter, agreed in September 2006 between the Council of Heads of Medical Schools and the BMA Medical Students Committee, sets out the responsibilities of medical students and university medical schools for the duration of the undergraduate period. Although not a legal document, the charter serves to promote a coherent relationship between students and their medical schools to help improve students' learning experiences.

Modernising Medical Careers

Modernising Medical Careers (MMC), implemented in 2005, is the initiative which provides the major reform of postgraduate medical education.

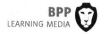

Following graduation in Medicine, a structured programme for the further training of junior doctors – broad based initially, and focusing upon specialisation later – means that patients can be assured that all doctors reach the required level of competency.

The MMC programme also ensures that doctors undergo regular and structured assessments of their skills. As the initiative develops, it is envisaged that these assessments will be conducted by senior doctors, such as consultants, and experienced healthcare professionals from outside Medicine, such as senior nursing staff.

The MMC format for postgraduate training comprises:

Foundation Year 1: This provides broad clinical experience in the first year following graduation from university.

Foundation Year 2: The junior doctor builds upon that first year's experience, with special focus on emergency care for patients.

It is during the course of these two years that junior doctors decide their chosen field of specialisation – in one of the many hospital based specialities, in public health, or in general practice.

One concern relating to the MMC format is that doctors may gain experience in some minor specialties, such as Histopathology, for example, for a very short period – perhaps even only one week as a 'taster' attachment.

The MMC reforms might, therefore, jeopardise recruitment to certain minor specialties.

After completing the two Foundation Years, there then follows:

Core Specialist Training: A two-year programme which provides introductory experience in the chosen specialty.

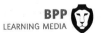

Higher Specialist Training: Experience gained during this period, which may extend up to around five years dependent upon the specialty, leads to the doctor becoming competent to become a consultant in the field, or a principal in general practice.

A certificate of completion of specialist training (CCST) is issued by the General Medical Council to doctors who have successfully completed a programme of Higher Specialist Training.

MMC website: www.mmc.nhs.uk

National Health Service

The NHS was established in 1948 in an attempt to make health services available to all citizens of the UK through a system dependent on public finance (from taxation and National Insurance) and publicly owned buildings. It sought to be universal in its coverage and comprehensive in terms of the services provided. The principle of equity of access on the basis of equal clinical need was enshrined in the structure of the NHS. In time, public finance has been supplemented by nominal charges for prescriptions, dental treatment and eye tests.

Issues for the NHS which remain are:

- **Resources:** in particular, the need to achieve equitable distribution and local flexibility.
- **Healthcare partnerships:** the increasing need to develop team and collaborative working between different groups of professionals, between primary care (GP) and hospital services, and between other authorities and agencies (such as social services and education).
- **Developing professional knowledge:** through training, research and audit, with a strong emphasis upon multi-disciplinary approaches.
- **Patient and carer involvement:** developing choice and recognising patients' rights AND their responsibilities.

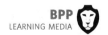

- **Better organisation:** through local linkages, managerial support and information technology.

NHS Constitution

For the first time in the history of the NHS, the Constitution presents details of what staff, patients and the public can expect from the National Health Service.

The Constitution also sets out the rights of NHS patients. These rights cover issues relating to:

- Access to health services
- The quality of care patients can expect, and
- The kinds of treatments which are available.

NHS Direct

NHS Direct is a service which delivers telephone and e-health information advice directly to the public throughout the 24-hour period.

The service seeks to provide information and advice about health, illness and health services, to enable patients and families to make decisions about their healthcare.

The telephone service aims to triage callers with disease symptoms so as then to be able to provide guidance on which healthcare organisation the caller should access.

Nurses working for NHS Direct are also able to give advice on how to manage an illness episode at home. Health Information Advisors can give information on a wide range of medical conditions and treatments, together with details of NHS policies and procedures. In some areas of the UK, the local Primary Care Trust commissions NHS Direct to provide the gateway for their out-of-hours GP cover arrangements.

NHS Direct began as a telephone health line in 1997; it now has a substantial health information website, including a comprehensive health encyclopaedia, and its own digital TV service. In 2010, almost five million patients used the NHS Direct telephone line, and nearly six million patients used the range of online health and symptom checkers.

NHS Direct website: www.nhsdirect.nhs.uk

National Institute for Health and Clinical Excellence (NICE)

NICE is the independent organisation responsible for providing national guidance on the promotion of good health and the prevention and treatment of ill health.

It was established to review clinical approaches with a specific aim of addressing the so-called 'postcode lottery' in which patients' access to established effective therapies can seemingly depend upon where they happened to live. Since 2005, the NHS in England and Wales has been legally obliged to provide funding for medicines and treatments recommended by NICE's technology appraisal board.

NICE formulates recommendations on the effectiveness and cost effectiveness of preventative and therapeutic approaches in three main areas:

- Public health: guidance on the promotion of good health and the prevention of ill health.
- Health technologies: guidance on the use of new and existing medicines, treatments and procedures conducted within the National Health Service.
- Clinical practice: guidance on the appropriate treatment and care of people with specific diseases and conditions by the NHS.

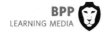

It is the Secretary of State for Health who requests NICE to review a particular technology or treatment. NICE then invites Consultee and Commentator organisations to carry out the appraisal.

Consultee organisations include patient groups, organisations representing healthcare professionals and the manufacturers of the product undergoing appraisal. Consultees submit evidence during the appraisal and comment upon the appraisal documents.

Commentator organisations include the manufacturers of products to which the technology undergoing appraisal is being compared. They comment upon the appraisal documents but do not actually submit information themselves.

An independent academic centre then draws together and analyses all of the published information relating to the technology under appraisal and prepares an assessment report. Comments are taken into account and changes made to the assessment report to produce an evaluation report. An independent Appraisal Committee then reviews the evaluation report and receives spoken testimony from clinical experts, patient groups and carers. An appraisal consultation document is then drawn up, and this is sent to all consultees and commentators for their further comments. The final appraisal determination document is then prepared, embracing all of these comments. This document is submitted to the board of NICE for approval.

NICE has set up several National Collaborating Centres which draw up the boundaries of the application of NICE's recommendations. The National Collaborating Centre then appoints a Guideline Development Group whose task it is to formulate guidelines for the application of the product in actual clinical practice.

Guideline Development Groups obtain their membership from healthcare professionals in the specific clinical field, and representatives of relevant patient and carer groups. The draft

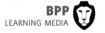

guideline is presented to stakeholder organisations who are invited to comment. An independent Guideline Review Panel ensures that these comments are fully considered; the Guideline Development Group then finalises the recommendations which are approved by NICE and issued to the NHS for adoption.

Fundamentally, the organisation's role is to determine how best to allocate the health service's limited resources.

Up until 2008, NICE had made their recommendations for the treatment of clinical conditions in line with the so called 'Rule of Rescue'.

The Rule of Rescue: this is the powerful human impulse to attempt to help an identifiable individual whose life is in danger on account of desperate or exceptional circumstances no matter how much it costs. NICE considers that when there are limited resources for healthcare, then to spend too much on one patient may deny others, and that applying the 'Rule of Rescue' may mean that other people will not have the care or treatment they need. NICE now state that saving a life could not be justified at any cost.

Currently, NICE does not normally sanction the use of a drug on the NHS above the cost figure of £30,000 per Quality Adjusted Life Year.

NICE 'do not do' database

In addition to providing recommendations upon good practice, NICE has also compiled a database of 'do not do' recommendations. These are clinical practices which should be discontinued completely or should not be used routinely, thus helping to reduce service inefficiencies.

NICE website: www.nice.org.uk

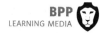

National Service Frameworks

National Service Frameworks are authoritative statements detailing:

- Clear quality standards for healthcare for certain groups of people, or for patients suffering from specific conditions; and
- Strategies to enable organisations achieve these standards.

National Service Frameworks are developed by health professionals, patients, carers and voluntary agencies working in partnership.

There are National Service Frameworks for:

- **Cancer** services
- **Mental health** services
- Services aimed at preventing and treating **coronary heart disease** and **strokes**
- **Older people**
- Services providing care for **children**
- Services providing care for patients with **diabetes**
- **Renal** services
- Services for people with **long term conditions**
- Services for patients with **chronic obstructive airways disease**

Organ donation

Transplant surgery has helped thousands of people. However, the gap between the number of people who would benefit from an organ transplant and the number who actually receive the organ has widened. Currently in the United Kingdom, people must positively sign up to the organ register – or their families agree – before their organs can be used.

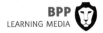

At the end of 2010 it was estimated that in the UK:

- Every day three people die while on the waiting list for transplant surgery.
- More than 8,000 people were waiting for transplant surgery, but only around 4,000 of these procedures are carried out each year.

Presumed consent

There is considerable support from amongst some politicians and clinicians for changing the law in the UK so that doctors could assume that someone who had died in an accident had consented for their remaining intact organs to be used for the benefit of others. Some countries, such as Spain and Belgium, already operate under a law of presumed consent. However, in the UK so far, calls for legal change have been resisted.

Pandemic

The World Health Organisation currently defines 'pandemic' as '...the worldwide spread of a new disease. An influenza pandemic occurs when a new influenza virus emerges and spreads around the world, and most people do not have immunity'.

Postcode lottery

It was in 1971 that *The Lancet* published a seminal article, *The Inverse Care Law* written by Dr Julian Tudor Hart. The author argued then that the availability of good medical care tended to vary inversely with the need for it in the population. He referred to lessons being learnt during the first fifteen years of the NHS, and in particular that there was variation:

- In the quality of medical specialist attention, and maternal care, and
- In rates of elective surgical procedures.

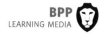

Reports indicating that people in some parts of the country may be denied an NHS treatment or a diagnostic test on account, seemingly, of where they live continue to be published.

A report from the Department of Health entitled *The Atlas of Variation* was published in November 2010. The report shows how primary care trusts across the country vary in their care of patients, their costs and their outcomes.

The Atlas shows:

- A 14-fold difference in spend on broken hips.
- A four-fold variation in the proportion of stroke patients who spend most of their time in a dedicated stroke unit.
- A 38-fold difference in rates of obesity surgery.

Some commentators have concluded that the report indicates that the sharing of good practice from one hospital to another is still not widespread across the NHS.

Primary Care Trusts

Primary care is the care provided by the health professionals normally seen when anyone first has a problem. It might be a visit to a GP, or a dentist, or optician for an eye test, or pharmacist to buy a hay fever medication. NHS Walk-in Centres, and NHS Direct are also primary care health services. Many of these services are managed by local NHS Primary Care Trusts (PCTs).

In addition to these management responsibilities, PCTS also **commission** the provision of local NHS care – this includes care provided by hospital services for local people.

PCTs work alongside Local Authority services, for example Social Services, and other agencies to make sure that local community needs are met in a co-ordinated manner. PCTs are in an excellent position to understand the health needs of the

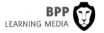

people they serve and ensure the effective provision of healthcare to the community.

Key doctors working in Primary Care Trusts are:

- Local General Practitioners, who are close to the people they care for and can listen carefully to their concerns.
- Specialists in public health, who are skilled in assessing the health needs of the public.

The Royal College of Physicians

The Royal College of Physicians is a registered charity which aims to ensure high quality care for patients by promoting the highest standards of medical practice. The college provides and sets standards in clinical practice and education and training, conducts assessments and examinations (including the examination for the Membership of the Royal College of Physicians), and quality assures clinical audit projects and programmes of such audits. The college also publishes bi-monthly a medical journal, *Clinical Medicine*, formerly named *The Journal of the Royal College of Physicians*.

The Royal College of Physicians also assures programmes of continuing professional development for all its members.

Other important Royal Colleges in the field of Medicine include the Royal College of Surgeons and the Royal College of General Practitioners.

Top-up treatments

One key founding principle of the publicly funded NHS is that patients are not provided with treatments that they want, but with what they need. Need for treatment is taken to mean ability to benefit from it; that is, the treatment must be effective. However, within scarce NHS resources, there is also the requirement for treatment to be cost-effective – to provide

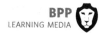

value for money. Meeting this requirement causes rationing of health service treatments.

In 2008, NICE decided not to recommend certain high cost cancer drugs on the grounds that they did not extend life by long enough to justify their cost: some of these treatments cost over £30,000 per year. Some patients sought to receive this treatment by paying for it themselves via private prescriptions. However, the ruling was that patients should receive their healthcare *either* entirely from the private sector or entirely from the NHS. This would have meant that if a patient obtained the high cost treatment privately, they would then have all their NHS care removed.

It became apparent during the autumn of 2008 that some patients receiving NHS care were indeed buying expensive cancer drugs unavailable on the NHS as dozens of hospital trusts exploited a logistical loop-hole. The rule is that private and NHS treatment cannot be mixed in the 'same episode of care'. Some hospital trusts were getting around this rule by having one doctor prescribe the NHS care element of a patient's treatment, and another doctor prescribing the drug privately, which counts as two separate episodes of care. Accordingly, a review was carried out, led by Professor Mike Richards, into how access to medicines for NHS patients might be improved. In 2009, and in the light of that review, the Department of Health published guidance which made clear that NHS patients should not lose their entitlement to NHS care as a result of choosing to buy additional private care.

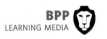

More titles in the Entry to Medical School Series

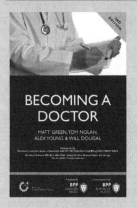

£14.99
October 2011
Paperback
978-1-445381-51-0

Deciding on whether or not to pursue a career in medicine is a decision that should not be taken lightly. Becoming a doctor can be highly rewarding but is not without its drawbacks. It is therefore important that you gain a clear insight into the world of medicine to ensure that it is the right path for you to follow.

This book has been written with the above in mind to provide a clear picture of what becoming a doctor really involves. In this comprehensive book Matt Green and Tom Nolan explore:

- What it really means to be a good doctor

- The steps that should be taken to confirm whether a career in medicine is really the one for you

- How to successfully apply to medical school including the various entrance exams (UKCAT, BMAT, GAMSAT), the UCAS personal statement and subsequent medical school interview

- Life as a student at medical school and how to excel

- The various career paths open to you as a doctor with invaluable insights provided by practising doctors.

This engaging and comprehensive book is essential reading for anyone serious about becoming a doctor and determining whether it really is the right career for you!

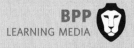

More titles in the Entry to Medical School Series

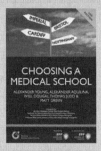

CHOOSING A MEDICAL SCHOOL

£19.99

December 2011

Paperback

978-1-445381-50-3

Choosing which Medical Schools to apply to is a decision that should not be taken lightly. It is important that you do your homework and consider carefully the many factors that differ between each institution.

This comprehensive and insightful guide written by medical students, for medical students, covers everything you need to know to enable you to select the Medical Schools best suited to you. The book is designed to help school leavers, graduates and mature individuals applying to Medical School, together with parents and teachers.

The first part of the book covers what to expect from life at medical school and things to consider prior to applying.

The second part then features chapters covering each individual UK Medical School. Each chapter is written by current medical students at the institution and is broken down into sections on the medical school, the university and the city finishing with the views of pre-clinical and clinical students.

This book is best used in conjunction with 'Becoming a Doctor'.

Key Features:

- **Forewords** - by Sir Liam Donaldson (Chief Medical Officer of England), Professor Ian Gilmore (President of Royal College of Physicians), Mr John Black (President of Royal College of Surgeons) and Professor Mike Larvin (Director of Education Royal College of Surgeons)

- **Insider Information** - An overview of what to expect from life at Medical School and tips for getting in and staying ahead

- **Latest Admission Statistics and Advice** - Up-to-date information on course structure, teaching methods, entrance requirements and other key factors to consider when choosing a Medical School

- **Pre-Medical and Postgraduate Advice** – views from preclinical and postgraduate students on getting in and what to consider

- **Easy Comparisons** - Quick comparison table covering each UK Medical School

- **Medical Education** - Clear sections focussing on pre-clinical and clinical education including summaries of teaching methods, support, examinations and teaching hospitals

- **Extracurricular Activities** - Information on what extracurricular opportunities are available at each Medical School and in the surrounding city

- **Students' Views** - Opinions and insights for each Medical School by current medical students

By using this engaging, easy to use and comprehensive guide, you will remove so much of the uncertainty surrounding how to best select the Medical Schools that are right for you.

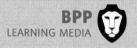

BPP LEARNING MEDIA

www.bpp.com/health

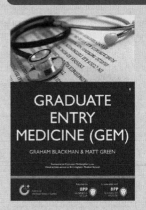
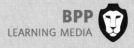

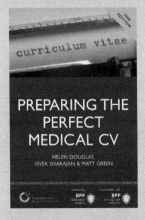
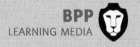

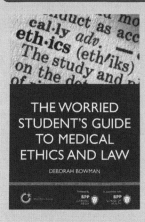
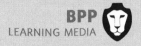

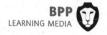